LIMS

Applied Information Technology
for the Laboratory

LIMS

Applied Information Technology
for the Laboratory

Richard R. Mahaffey

VNR VAN NOSTRAND REINHOLD
_____ New York

Library of Congress Catalog Card Number 89-31192
ISBN 0-442-31820-0

Printed in the United States of America

Van Nostrand Reinhold
115 Fifth Avenue
New York, New York 10003

Van Nostrand Reinhold International Company Limited
11 New Fetter Lane
London EC4P, 4EE, England

Van Nostrand Reinhold
480 La Trobe Street
Melbourne, Victoria 3000, Australia

Nelson Canada
1120 Birchmount Road
Scarborough, Ontario M1K 5G4, Canada

16 15 14 13 12 11 10 9 8 7 6 5 4 3 2 1

Library of Congress Cataloging-in-Publication Data

Mahaffey, Richard R., 1950-
    LIMS : applied information technology for the laboratory / Richard
R. Mahaffey.
        p.   cm.
    Includes index.
    ISBN 0-442-31820-0
    1. Laboratories—Management—Data processing.   2. Management
information systems.   I. Title.
Q183.A1M34   1989
507′.8—dc19   89-31192
                                                           CIP

Preface

Computing and information management technologies touch our lives in the environments where we live, play and, work. High tech is becoming the standard. Those of use who work in a laboratory environment are faced with an obvious challenge. How do we best apply these technologies to make money for our companies? The first level of deliverable benefits is achieved through task automation. The second level is obtained by integrating the individual islands of automation. The third, or top level, of benefits is related to applying intelligence to computing applications.

The use of computing technology, at level one, to automate lab procedures, methods, and instruments has been profitable for many years. We can easily find yearly returns in the range of 10-50% for investments at this level. For level two, the integration of some applications has evolved and has led to data management systems and local area networking in the lab environment. Investment paybacks at level two are substantially higher, in the range of 200-400%. Examples of applications at the top level, that of intelligent systems and applications, are few and far between. And what about the payback for investments at this level? With such limited experience at level three, we can only estimate the benefits. But again, they appear to be much higher, in the range of 2000-4000%.

Unfortunately, there are no quantum leaps between these levels. The question thus becomes, how do we bridge the gaps? Laboratory Information Management Systems (LIMS) can provide these bridges in a laboratory environment. A LIMS provides a mechanism not only to build automated tasks but to integrate them as well. Thus, the bridge between levels one and two is apparent. With the imaginative use of LIMS and the development of imaginative features by LIMS vendors, we can reach level three. The developers of LIMS are doing a great job. Our purchases will encourage the vendors, of course, but we still need to communicate needs and new ideas to them routinely. The analytical community has spawned this new LIMS market, and it is our responsibility to nurture it. If we want new laboratory products to facilitate automation and information management, such as a standard computer interface for all laboratory instruments, we must not fail to speak out. The time is right. The vendors are listening.

The primary purpose of this book is to further the understanding of

LIMS, and to explain why they are needed and what they are. It is suggested reading for anyone preparing to purchase LIMS software, the laboratory member planning to write LIMS software, the vendor/developer of LIMS software, the laboratory member or manager who seeks more efficient lab operations and wants a better understanding of LIMS, and the college chemistry student (bachelor and above) interested in gaining more knowledge about the concept of laboratory information management.

This book is divided into five sections. Section One describes some fundamental concepts of laboratory information. LIMS is our avenue to the future, but by understanding where we've been and where we are now, the future becomes much closer. Sections Two and Three describe what LIMS are made of and how to choose and manage a LIMS. Section Four deals with getting the most out of the LIMS investment and the related concepts of computer systems validation and LIMS justification. Section Five presents some futuristic views of LIMS functions and applications.

Every aspect of contemporary information technology is undergoing rapid change, and LIMS is no exception. By the time this writing is in print, at least two of the LIMS packages used herein to provide descriptive examples will have undergone substantial change. One package will no longer be offered, and the author of another package will have announced the intention of discontinuing business as an original LIMS software manufacturer.

Our imaginations are our only limitations in computer applications! And I hope you too believe that computerizing the laboratory is no exception. It is my firm belief that LIM also stands for "Laboratory IMagination."

Contents

Section One

Laboratory Information Concepts

Chapter 1

Introduction to Laboratory Information Management

Information, with its antecedents and all its associated concepts, is the most all-encompassing, most influential force in human existence. The following chapters deal with managing a particular type of information. This information, although scientific for the most part, is really no different from any other form of information. It is collected, stored, and used — with some amount being discarded quickly, some kept for a finite time period, and some retained forever. When we need information that is not available, new technologies are developed to obtain it. To develop the new technologies, more information is needed. This process creates an ever-enlarging information spiral. The more information we have, the more information we need.

Because information is so important to us and because its management is not a simple task, we will make a cursory examination of information and some related concepts. This will help to reinforce our basic understanding of information and its value.

Information, Knowledge, Intelligence, Experience

Since the Pleistocene Period, and for a wide variety of reasons, the quest for knowledge and information has directed our fate. Information about food and predators meant survival to early man. Galileo's pure desire for knowledge resulted in his condemnation but set the stage for modern astronomy. Bohr's disputed theory on the structure of the atom was considered almost insignificant at the time, but subseqently led to a focus of information development in Oak Ridge, and in other locations, that resulted in the atomic bomb. For the sheer desire to be first, Watson and Crick, who elucidated the structure of DNA, stretched the limits of science to discover new information. A political promise that Americans would walk on the moon by the end of the 1960s launched an information gathering effort second to none in history, and resulted in an order of magnitude increase in computer technology.

Not only does everyone need different types of information to live and work, but the information required is constantly changing. As each day passes, additional information is discovered. Some of it is learned or stored, and some is rejected. In most cases, the new information does not replace old information; it is simply added. How much information does the brain hold? Let's assume that a person 40 years old has learned an average of one page of information per day. A page of text can be stored on a computer in an average of 4000 bytes. Using computer storage equivalence to estimate 40 years of information storage, the person has stored the equivalent of 58.4 megabytes. If U.S. population is 225 million, with an average age of 40, we have over 13 million gigabytes of information.

Of course, these estimates are silly, but they do enable us to visualize the overwhelming amount of information around us. It is important to us and our employers to understand the value of information. New information will always exist. The methods by which we select the information we want, store it, and use it ultimately mean the difference between our successes and failures. Before we consider the value of information further, let's see what *information* really is by comparing it with three related terms — *knowledge, intelligence,* and *experience*.

A person gains information from experience, experimentation, trial and error, reading, listening, etc. Conscious, human adult activity, with a few exceptions, is based on information. We brush our teeth because we have information about the consequences of not brushing. Although we may never have been stung by a hornet, we don't move a hornet's nest from a tree branch because we have information that getting stung hurts. In the previous sentences we could easily substitute the word *knowledge* for *information* and still convey the same message. Does this mean that information is knowledge, and vice versa? Or have we applied some information, or knowledge, and somehow unconsciously equated the two? Webster's Dictionary (59) provides the following definitions:

Information — 1. something told; news; intelligence; word.
                2. knowledge acquired in any manner; facts; data; learning; lore.
                3. any data that can be stored in and retrieved from a computer.

Knowledge — acquaintance with facts; range of information, awareness, or understanding.

Intelligence — the ability to learn or understand from experience; ability to acquire and retain knowledge.

Experience — knowledge, skill, or practice resulting from (activity that includes training, observation of practice, and personal participation).

Thus, information, knowledge, intelligence, and experience are without a doubt interrelated, and, to answer the above question, the words *information* and *knowledge* are the same in some instances. But there are some important differences and points which should be examined. To have knowledge about some subject certainly means to have information about it. Having knowledge also implies having a relatively large quantity of information. This quantity measure is evident in the "range of information" and "understanding" components of the above definition of knowledge. We also note that the definition of intelligence says nothing about applying knowledge, only gaining and retaining it. Experience, however, does include application and practice. It also connotes having knowledge, which we have stated means having a great deal of information. But the concept of experience has no measure of quality. For example, if we know that a dog trainer has trained hundreds of dogs, we can say without hesitation that this trainer is experienced. But have the dogs learned anything? Does experience make a good trainer? Not necessarily.

The point of these comparisons is twofold:

1. Merely having information, knowledge, intelligence, and experience, is of no value by itself. The value of these concepts obviously comes from their use. We can hire the most knowledgeable and intelligent engineer on the face of the planet, but if the engineer doesn't produce, what good is she or he to the company? We may install a $10M computer system with a 100 gigabyte database of competitor product information, but if its never used, what is it worth?
2. Information is the basis of knowledge, intelligence, and experience. It is the all-important foundation for everything we do from staying alive to using intelligence against our business competitors.

The Value of Information

How can we put a value on information? Assume that we purchased a dictionary, with 1700 pages of information, for $30. Is the value of the information contained in the dictionary $30? Suppose that we needed to

send a letter to a client who not only is an avid bird-watcher and or-
nithologist, but who is a linguist and demands correct spelling. In trying
our best to be cordial in the hope of making a sale, we mentioned a
family of grosbeak birds which have nested in a tree outside our window.
Thinking the spelling might be *grossbeak,* we used the $30 dictionary to
obtain the correct spelling, sent the letter, which was very well received,
and made a $30,000 sale. Suppose that misspelling the word *grosbeak*
had resulted in a loss of the sale; was the value of the information $30
or $30,000? Clearly the value of the dictionary is still $30 (less depre-
ciation), but the information it contains obviously has a different value.
The value of information, therefore, is not related to the cost of obtaining
the information, but rather to its use.

How Much Information Do We Need?

Again, we do not benefit from merely having information; the only benefit
comes from using it. Then, does it follow that the more information we
have, the more we can potentially benefit? Maybe and maybe not. For
example, if we need to buy some computer terminals, is it necessary to
obtain quotations from all terminal vendors in order to determine a good
price? If we're interested in knowing how many batches out of 1000 we
can expect to be out of specs, is it necessary to run 1000 batches to find
out? The answer to both questions is obviously no. If we want to find
the best hot dog maker in New York City, will we need more than 10
samples? If we want to know who in the world could afford a takeover
of our company, do we need more than a representative sample? The
answer to these two questions is yes. Thus, sometimes it will be very
hard to acquire enough information. At other times, we can calculate in
advance how much information we need. And at still other times, we
won't know how much information we need until we have it.

It is widely accepted that information is as much an asset to a company
as any capital item. Decisions based on data and knowledge are certainly
more likely to be correct. But these are not new ideas. Information has
always been the life blood of corporations. A Japanese industry leader
stated that American industry has no chance of catching up in quality
production for one primary reason: Corporate management makes all the
decisions, and the uninvolved workers carry them out. Thus, it's no
wonder quality suffers. And, until quite recently, at least, it has been
true. Today, U.S. corporate management philosophies are changing. Decisions are being made at lower levels. Team management is replacing
the organizational hierarchy. Organizations are being streamlined and
flattened. Everyone in the organization knows that everyone is responsible for quality.

Management Trends and Information

Do these management trends have an effect on information? Very much so. Such trends mean that more and more people are depending on information; information flows must therefore broaden to accommodate the increasing demand. Trusting employees' decisions will certainly be easier if management knows that they are based on information and data. However, getting the right information to the right people at the right time is the main problem. Fortunately, we have some tools which will help us solve these problems. They are machines used for information management. They can be purchased from manufacturers such as Apple, Cray, DEC, HP, IBM, PE, Prime, Unisys, and others.

Information and Quality

If we get the right information to the right people at the right time, what should they do with it? Assuming that these people are our employees, we hope that they will use it to sustain a commitment to quality. Quality cannot be "built into" a product. When we hear people say that they have done so, we should be alarmed. A product is either a quality product or it isn't. If any part of a product's development and manufacture is left to chance or built without supporting information, it is not a quality product. Quality is not a feature; it is a state which can only be obtained by having the right information at the right time, regardless of the cost.

Designing a product correctly the first time and building it the same way repeatedly ensures quality. Testing a product does not somehow implant quality. No amount of testing will change the quality. Do we want a car that is advertised as being subjected to several hundred tests after manufacture to ensure quality, or do we want a car that's built so well that it doesn't need to be tested later? There is a difference. The difference is in the attitude toward quality. If a manufacturer thinks that quality can be bought or added as an afterthought, the quality will be low.

Quality manufacturing means less testing. Less testing means less expense. Quality manufacturing means fewer complaints, fewer returns, and more satisfied customers. This can only be achieved by gathering information, gaining knowledge, and applying intelligence to planning, engineering, design, manufacture, and marketing. Quality starts with information.

Dependence on Laboratory Information

In a manufacturing organization, much of the business is based on laboratory information. Production control laboratories pace output and can even shut down production based on laboratory information. Cost and budget estimates for new product development depend on laboratory information. Capacity and personnel plans are based on predictions of new product development. Customer complaints often result in the generation of laboratory information. Although it may only be a small percentage of the total information generated, information from the laboratory is one of the most important types.

Laboratory information is showcased in technical and innovation reports and in the scientific literature. It invariably shows up in patent applications and federal regulation compliance documentation. Government and commercial testing facilities have the production of laboratory information as their sole output and their reason for being. Clinical laboratory information is used to diagnose illness and save lives. Can anything be more important than that?

Why Do We Need to Manage Laboratory Information?

American industry is being pressured as never before to shorten new product development times. The time from idea to innovation to prototype, and finally to market, must be reduced in order to increase market share relative to foreign competition. As scientists in research laboratories struggle to reduce delay, they must cope with an equally devastating problem — product quality. Finally, compliance with Good Laboratory Practices (GLP) and federal regulations place minimum analytical requirements at a very high level.

We appear to be balancing on a double edged sword. If we sacrifice quality, our products won't sell. If we're late getting them to market, they won't sell. What can members of analytical laboratories do to help? An opportunity is at hand. A focus on the quality of laboratory data has become a means of attacking some of our problems. For example, if lab members reduce the need to retest samples by doing them right the first time, or reduce the need for duplicate samples by earning our customers' trust, then they have made a significant contribution to reducing the number of samples and speeding up development. If they can increase sample throughput, reduce turnaround times, and at the same time increase output quality, they have again made a significant contribution.

The way to maintain high quality laboratory data is to make sure that laboratory processes are in control. We must give scientists tools with which to gain the most information possible from the fewest number of samples in the least amount of time. Information management is a process which needs to be controlled. The use of a Laboratory Information Management System (LIMS), properly implemented, provides an efficient means to control the information management process in order to get the most out of the data.

Managing Change in the Laboratory

Change must be managed in all areas of business, and the laboratory is no exception. In our laboratories, analysts, chemists, engineers, other scientists, management, and customers all change with time as promotions are earned and retirements occur. Samples, test methods, and expectations all change. The internal and external rules and regulations by which we operate change. Changes in raw materials, instrumentation, and computer systems are inevitable.

Writers of management theory all warn that change is the number one enemy of business (6–9). Russell Ackoff (6) states that "companies and governments are going out of business every day because they have failed to adapt to [change] or have adapted too slowly." And fueling the change is a less predictable, larger environment of "increasing inter-connectedness and interdependence of individuals, groups, organizations, institutions, and societies brought about by changes in communications and transportation." Donald Schon (9) tells us that change is accelerating, problems are becoming more complex, the problems that face us are changing more rapidly all the time, and that by the time we find solutions to many problems, the solutions aren't "relevant or effective."

The best way to manage change in any business sector is, first, to have a system in place which is strong and flexible enough to be adapted to change. The system should also be required to collect data on itself and to provide information whereby changes can be monitored. A LIMS, properly implemented, can not only withstand the environmental changes to which it is subjected, but can also help the laboratory as a whole to withstand change. A LIMS can easily manage data by exception. It can be programmed to maintain counts of samples for different analytical methods, thus providing the data from which predictive assumptions can be derived. It can schedule work, people, and instruments, bill for work done, fill out time cards, maintain statistics, and alert someone only when there is a problem.

A New Computer Application Technology Is Born

Automation in the laboratory is not new (3). The past 20 years have seen an explosive growth in the application of electronics in the laboratory. Today's new instruments make measurements faster and better than ever before, and they practically run themselves. With each new instrument generation our laboratories become more efficient; hopefully, this trend will never end.

Gigabytes of computer program code have been written in the past 10 years to process and manage laboratory data. Data systems, including hardware, have evolved as well. Today's new laboratory systems combine instrument and data management software, and layer attractive graphics applications on top.

A recent "Buyers Guide" (5) lists 23 "Lab Database Management" application packages. Seven years ago, how many packages would have been on this list? About 10. So, computer programs for laboratory data management are hardly new. But then, what is?

What is new is the realization, of software vendors that there is a new application technology ready to be explored and developed. Those of us working in laboratories for the past 15 years have known that it was coming, and in fact have written our own bits and pieces of it. The application of computers to the management of all information centered in our laboratories is now becoming a reality. We have witnessed the birth of this realization and should deem it the beginning of a new application technology.

Approximately 20 dedicated LIMS are now commercially available, compared to 1 or 2 in 1980. A few of these new systems have made their way out of corporate laboratories, and others are provided by long-lived laboratory data product vendors. Vendors, for their own survival, try to be responsive to their customers' needs. We chemists and laboratory support systems analysts can take pride that we are responsible for this new application technology. We have worked with the vendors, telling them what we have needed for years. We have brought them into our laboratories and shown them what they could do for us.

What Is Laboratory Information?

The output of every laboratory is information. A thorough understanding of laboratory processes yields the knowledge of what information is important. In most laboratories, the manager will be the person most familiar with all of the laboratory's processes, and therefore should know most about its information. Should we expect to have an absolute definition of *laboratory information?* Let's look at some reduced raw data. A three-question survey was given to a group of lab managers in a physical and analytical chemistry services division of the Eastman Kodak Company. The questions and a synopsis of the responses are listed below. Many of the responses were very similar. They were combined and grouped as neatly as possible for presentation here. Several exact quotes were used for emphasis and are enclosed in quotations marks.

1. What does "laboratory information" mean to you?
    Responses: a. Test results, data, interpretations
               b. Records of sample receipt and status

  c. Records of analysis (who, when, what)
  d. Instrument performance records
   Control charts
   Calibrations
   Maintenance
  e. Documented laboratory outputs
  f. Reports, graphs, tables
  g. Answers to questions
  h. Routine data obtained from tests

2. What does "management of laboratory information" mean to you?
 Responses: a. The provision, maintenance, and use of a system providing for the entering, modification, archiving, transferring, statistical analysis, and retrieving of data and laboratory information.
    b. The planning, directing, organizing, and control of laboratory outputs in order to fulfill the company's mission.
    c. Handling data, interpretations, and results in an organized way so that the people who require it, have it when they need it.

3. Use your imagination and describe the "perfect" LIMS.
 Responses: a. Response time is fast (This answer appeared on nearly every response.)
    b. User friendly:
     Minimum number of menus involved
     Minimize number of times sample number must be entered; "bar coding will probably solve this problem"
    c. Control sample data transferred automatically from LIMS to statistical spreadsheet; "this will save 400 man-hours per year"
    d. "Our customers [internal] will all be using LIMS to receive their data. It will have to be easy for them to use LIMS if we expect them to do so."
    e. Handle all paperwork
    f. Provide summary information — trends, samples run, turnaround time, information on customers, etc.
    g. "Make it easy to adhere to standards (gentle but insistent)"
    h. "Should be smarter than I am about getting useful statistics about stored information"
    i. Perform input/output to any "normal" device
    j. Easy to ask nonstandard questions

The above survey responses are summaries of actual responses. Let's further summarize the responses for each question:

1. What does "laboratory information" mean?
   — Documented test results, control charts, data, interpretations, graphs, instrument performance, records of analysis.
2. What does "management of laboratory information" mean?
   — The use of a "system" for management, planning, organizing, control of laboratory outputs, statistical analysis, archival, organized method of having information available when needed.
3. What is the "perfect" LIMS?
   — Fast, user friendly, automatic data transfer, bar coding, paperless, provide summary information about samples and customers, device independent, provides trends, statistics, standards.

We take a close look at many of the components of laboratory information in Chapter 2, but in general, it centers on production of test results. The purpose for managing laboratory information is twofold:

1. To have information readily available for those who need it.
2. To allow planning of all laboratory functions.

It may be argued that these two purposes are aspects of the same function and that all information we collect about anything is used for planning. But we'll leave that issue for others to ponder.

Requirements for a LIMS

The requirements for a LIMS, from an implementation standpoint, are fairly well defined. From above, the following can be considered requirements:

Fast, user friendly, automatic data transfer, bar coding, paperless, provides summary information about samples and customers, device independent, provides trends, statistics, standards.

None of these requirements are trivial. Each is a substantial concept. Although no existing system perfectly incorporates all of them as standard features, such a system will soon be a reality. (Chapter 16 presents future considerations related to LIMS.) These concepts are, for the most part, very simple, and without doubt possible with today's technology. LIMS have been evolving and will continue to evolve. Systems will come and go. In-house written systems will make it to market and go public. As the requirements we have defined here become commonplace, new and exciting features and products not even dreamed about will also become requirements.

Summary

In this chapter, we looked at some of the simple requirements for a LIMS. We viewed LIMS as a means to control the laboratory information management process in order to maintain high quality laboratory data. We reported that new interest in integrated management of all laboratory information is the beginning of a new application technology. It is hard to imagine the magnitude of accomplishments that we will see in the laboratory in the next 10 years. The blending of instrument, computer, and information management technologies will redefine the standards for laboratory performance. Total commitment to electronic notebooks and paperless laboratories is no longer just a vision of research directors. It is within our grasp.

Chapter 2

Laboratories, Laboratory Information, Computers

In Chapter 1 we examined the value of information. In Chapter 3 we will consider laboratory automation in terms of laboratory information management. The purpose of this chapter is to review some concepts and definitions, as well as future considerations of information management in the laboratory. Considerations which are important to information management in this environment are laboratories, laboratory information, and computers.

Laboratories

Laboratories whose sole purpose is to perform controlled tests on samples, exist under a variety of names such as *analytical, control, production control, physical testing, quality assurance,* and *materials testing laboratories.* These laboratories may differ immensely in size, complexity, instrumentation, automation, etc., but they have several similarities related to samples processing:

1. Samples are usually not generated in the laboratories; instead, they are delivered.
2. Testing produces results (data) which must be delivered outside the laboratory.
3. The laboratory's customers want results as soon as possible.
4. Information concerning similar samples is similar.
5. Samples are somehow tracked through the laboratory.
6. Counts of sample throughput are maintained to assist in resource allocation, budgeting, and billing.

Other laboratories, such as some research laboratories, differ only in that they may produce and analyze their own samples, with the test results used internally. Thus, the lab personnel are their own customers when it comes to analyzing samples. Maintaining sample counts is probably not necessary because the lab's output is not related to the number of samples processed.

Physical and analytical testing laboratories all have another factor in common: They are in a constant state of change. New models of instruments are announced regularly. New models are purchased either to add capacity and capability or to replace old units. Employees earn promotions and move out, they retire, and they quit. But regardless of their reason for leaving, the result is the same — change. Job openings are filled by either transferring personnel internally or hiring from the outside. New employees have different skills. The rules and regulations which govern day-to-day operations change. The only thing that is consistent about lab operation over a 1- to 2-year period is change. But even the rate of change is increasing, mostly due to advances in computing technology.

"Computers, robotics, and networks may or may not play a role in your laboratory at the moment, but there is no doubt that they will in the very near future" (37). Let's try to imagine a laboratory in the year 2000, or even 1995. How do we predict samples will be handled? How many instruments will print out results which must be manually entered into the LIMS? Will there be a LIMS in every laboratory? It is difficult for some of us to imagine operating a lab without taking advantage of the latest computing technology. By the year 2000, all laboratories will be making effective use of computing. This is said with almost complete certainty, because if they aren't, they won't be in business.

The laboratory manager must be able to manage the changes that the laboratory is facing. Coping with change is a major responsibility and time requirement for the manager. A potential danger is apparent. The application of computing technology to all phases of lab operation is in full swing, and all signs indicate that we can expect this trend to continue. We must make sure that laboratory managers embrace computing technology and strive to become leaders in implementation and promotion. A manager who is inclined to resist change might resist the inclusion of a new computer-based technology, and this tendency is dangerous. Time lost in the computing renaissance which our labs are undergoing equates to a loss of experience which can never be recovered. The efficiency of our laboratories cannot be jeopardized by the mismanagement of change.

Staffing laboratories with information systems specialists is becoming commonplace. Computing support staff from within the laboratory who report directly to lab management will be needed in the future. Laboratory computing cannot be managed from a central corporate Information Services (IS) department. The experience, needs, and goals of the laboratory are too diverse to guarantee a high percentage of correct decisions with this arrangement. Correct decisions concerning laboratory computing come from experience, from having a feel for the laboratory's overall responsibilities, and from being totally responsible to laboratory management. This isn't to say that central IS should be excluded. In fact, "the primary responsibility for the formation of strategies lies with the laboratory personnel and management, but it should be done in conjunction with corporate computer groups" (37). Their support is always needed in the areas of networks and compatibility.

A laboratory is one unit of a larger organization. The product of physical and analytical testing laboratories is information. A sample, accompanied by a small amount of sample information, comes into a testing lab. The sample is then converted into additional information. Compared to the amount of information entering the lab, the amount produced is many times greater. Links between different labs and between labs and other organizational units exist for one purpose: information flow. As we work to implement new technologies in our labs in order to produce more information faster, we must also consider the information flows into and out of the lab. A communications bottleneck will develop if we increase the amount of information produced in a lab over time without also increasing the amount coming out. Communication mechanisms designed to provide a more efficient and faster method of delivering the lab's information product are as important as the automation tools themselves.

Laboratory Information

Laboratory needs, functions, and other circumstances dictate which information is important. Labs which operate under the guidelines of federal regulatory agencies seem to maintain more data per sample than other labs. For example, raw data are usually retained for Food and Drug Administration (FDA) test validation proposals. In many other cases, only calculated results are retained. But test result data are only a small portion of the data managed by an analytical or physical testing laboratory. The total amount of information is tremendous. The following is a list of information which may be required or produced for every sample, analyst, and instrument (for definitions, see Appendix B):

Aliquot ID	Backlog trend
Analyst test certification	Calculated results
Archive history	Calculation algorithms
Audit trail	Charge number
Backlog	Comments by analyst

Comments by submitter
Date analyzed
Date approved
Date drawn
Date due
Date received
Error flags
Instrument calibration history
Instrument control limits
Instrument maintenance history
Number of samples per analyst
Number of samples per instrument
Oldest sample in lab
Project priority
Raw data
Required tests
Result limits
Result report destination
Result report format
Result validation and
  approval
Retain data date
Run number
Safety processing
  factors
Sample origin
Sample owner
Sample priority
Sample tracking
Sample type
Standard cost of test
Test limits
Turnaround time
Turnaround time trend
Unique sample ID

Clearly, there are many pieces of information which someone in the lab must manage. Are there more kinds of information now than in the past? A list of information produced 10-15 years ago would look similar, if not identical. Has anything changed concerning laboratory information? Absolutely! The number of these information items that we are now attempting to manage has increased. In the past, many of these types of information were not managed because manual methods of keeping the data were just too time consuming. The need to deliver test results was greater than the need to manage many types of information. Even instrument calibration and standard method validation were not done, or were done infrequently. Today instrument management is recognized as important. Federal regulatory guidelines, as described in Chapter 14, require the management of more of these types of information, and rightly so. The quality of the information produced by our analytical and physical testing labs is becoming an organizational strength. Through advances in instrumentation and automation, the number of samples being analyzed per analyst has dramatically increased. The absolute amount of data being produced has doubled over the past 10 years. Thus, we are managing more types of information than ever before, and the amount of information within each type is increasing.

The time has long since passed when laboratory analysts could manage all the required information with manual methods (38). The use of computer systems to manage pieces of laboratory information has been commonplace for many years. Computer programs to calculate results, maintain databases of test results, print reports, and produce control charts have long been integral components of laboratories. But how have we managed backlogs, instrument calibration histories, audit trails, and many of the other types of information? By manual methods. Today, however, we can no longer expect laboratory analysts to manage any information by manual methods. They can't keep up.

As we stated in Chapter 1, LIMS is providing the opportunity to apply computing technology to the management of all laboratory information. A LIMS, properly implemented, is an extremely valuable asset to an analytical or physical testing laboratory. "LIMS gives you a visibility of the operation of your lab that you never dreamed of before. You know how many samples failed, how many were done by each analyst or for a particular project" (35). It provides the means by which analysts can maintain control of the information they are required to manage. LIMS provides the method by which laboratories can process more and more samples by acting as a platform on which to build laboratory automation. It provides a path for future growth in both numbers of samples and quality of output.

Computers

Computers and Laboratory Communications

Development, over the past few years, of single-user personal computers (PCs) has reduced the cost of multifunction processing power, resulting in the appearance of many PC-based laboratory instruments. Multifunction processing is, of course, what PCs are all about. They can be used to perform a great variety of functions. The computing power of laboratory instrumentation has kept pace. As the cost of building computer circuitry into lab instruments decreases, their price/performance ratio declines. Less expensive, more sophisticated circuitry brings us better instruments for our money; however, it is the application of the multifunction PCs in laboratories that enables interfacing and data collection/processing with almost any make and model of instrument. Thus, the use of PCs in laboratories has become widespread. Laboratory instruments are complemented and enhanced by the use of an attached PC. In many cases, instruments are designed with a required PC connection.

It was noted in 1984 (33) that the historical development of laboratory devices and communications had proceeded in four phases. The next phase, phase five, was also predicted. The five phases are listed below. The accompanying dates indicate the approximate lifetime of the phase, and, of course, some phases haven't yet ended. These dates reflect periods of widespread use in analytical laboratories, not isolated usage in advanced (or lagging) laboratories. The development phases are:

1. *Manual data entry (1960–1975)* — Data are keypunched onto cards or paper tape and entered into the computer.
2. *Analog to digital (A/D) in the host (1970–1980)* — Laboratory devices are connected directly to the data processing system, which provides both control for the A/D controller and processing of the data.
3. *Digital to host (1975–1990)* — A/D conversion is done in the laboratory devices, with BCD or ASCII characters sent to the host computer.
4. *Intelligent lab devices (1980–????)* — Laboratory devices contain central processing units (CPUs) and preprocess data before sending them to the host computer.
5. *Multiple CPUs and intelligent devices on the network (1987–????)* — Local area networks of laboratory devices will develop using Ethernet and other technologies.

It was also noted in 1984 that "the personal computer may have come along too late for many instruments [and that] they will use chips instead" (33). This means that instruments would develop with sufficient intelligence and capability not only to process data but also to communicate directly with the host as a network device, which is the essence of the predicted phase five. As stated above, the inclusion of computer technology in lab instrumentation is commonplace. But what has occurred in the last few years in computer-to-instrument communications? The inclusion of networking components, including both hardware and software, in lab instruments has not happened. Instead, there has been a proliferation of PCs connected to all kinds of instruments, with networking of the PC becoming more popular.

Networking in the analytical lab is not new. Forms of networking were evident in the 1970s. The parallel General Purpose Instrument Bus (GPIB), also known by the names *IEEE-488 Bus* and *HP-IB Bus* (42), as well as HP's serial data loop chromatography systems, are networks in that they contain addressable devices and multiple instruments share the same communication path. These interface types are still in use.

Although networking components such as ethernet controllers have not been included in laboratory instruments, we are beginning to see the connection of instrumentation to the local area network using terminal servers. These instruments communicate like a terminal over the network and appear to the host computer and network as a dumb terminal. We are also beginning to see instruments connected to network servers specifically designed for lab instrumentation, such as network chromatography servers. These servers provide the network connection without having the actual network hardware/software within the instrument.

Information Management and Computers

Figure 2-1 illustrates the tools used for information management by analytical scientists over three decades, from the 1960s to the 1990s. The relative percentage of analytical scientists using each tool as their primary method is shown. Before 1980, the primary method of information management was by manual means. The maintenance of laboratory notebooks was an art. The use of paper filing systems, microfilm, and microfiche filing systems was a religion. Laboratory management was condemned if there were no such systems in place for information management and archival purposes. Before 1980, we saw the rise and fall of batch punched cards as a main computer method of information management. Only about 20% of analytical scientists used this method as their primary means of information management.

The primary method used by analytical scientists shifted from mostly manual methods to computer methods around 1980. By 1985, the multiuser minicomputer was by far the most popular computer tool for information management. This doesn't mean that laboratory notebooks are not being kept. They are, but only because laboratory guidelines, for legal reasons, require them. Most analytical scientists are using computer methods as their primary means of information management, which includes storage, search and retrieval, archiving, presentation, and transfer.

The multiuser minicomputer will continue to increase in use and will remain the primary tool for most analytical scientists throughout the 1990s. Multiuser software, compared to single-user workstation software, has already started to gain ground in usefulness and friendliness. Multiuser software will continue to improve, becoming the driving force behind the continued rise of the minicomputer. Use of the single-user, stand-alone workstation as the primary tool by analytical scientists, will peak in the early 1990s. These workstations will be networked to each other or to the department minicomputer, and thus won't be considered stand-alone technology. It is hard to envision how networked workstation technology will evolve beyond 1995. It is certain that the lifetime of the dumb terminal is nearing its end. (Terminals with built-in graphics capabilities aren't dumb.) The use of networked, diskless, graphics workstations is certain to increase, thus requiring a host as a server, which in most cases will be a minicomputer.

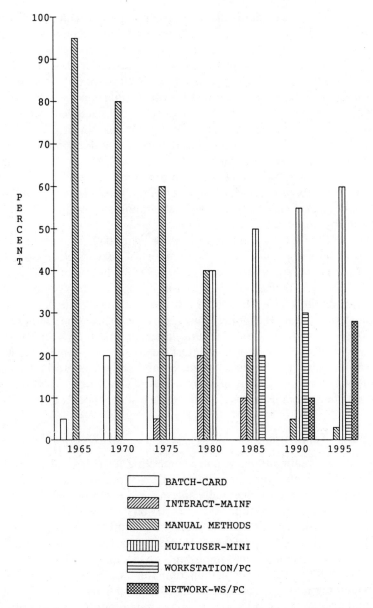

Figure 2-1. Primary information management tools used by analytical scientists.

In the 1970s, it was hardware that sold computers. During the 1980s, this situation changed. It is now software that sells computers. A prime example is the Apple Macintosh. The Mac does graphics very well, due mainly to incorporated graphics hardware. But other PCs can also do graphics well, so the hardware really isn't that special. It's the Mac software that is making it more and more popular and successful. The software gives the Mac an ease of use which is unequaled. Many of us know what an operating system is. We know the VMS, CMS, UNIX, and DOS operating systems. We know how to use them, we know their command syntax, and we generally know how they work. How many of us even know the name of the Mac operating system? How many of us with Macs even care what the operating system is called or how it works? We never see the operating system, and we certainly don't have to learn any command syntax.

What will the workstation be like in the year 2000? Will it even exist? It is very likely that some form of computer will take its place, something that most of us cannot even conceive. In 1978, how many of us could describe the Sun 4, E&S P300, Tektronix 4192, or VAXstation (on the high end) or the PC or Macintosh (on the low end)? Will the successor to this workstation technology have parallel processing, hundreds of megabytes of memory, and a natural language interface with voice recognition? Will the screen or user interface consist of a three-dimentional holographic display? It's hard to guess, and few of us are in a position to know — for sure. One thing is certain: Computer evolution is an exciting phenomenon to watch and be part of, even as a user.

Computer Applications

In the coming years, more and more computing activities will move closer to the user, away from the central CPU. Word processing, graphics processing, and even numerically intensive computing will be increasingly done on the desktop. As workstations become more powerful, laboratories will acquire them in increasing numbers for both dedicated and general-purpose applications. However, as stated above, multiuser computers will remain very important to the analytical scientist. The importance of the departmental minicomputer as a database, data sharing, and data integration platform is already well established. The dependence on rapid access to operational data is becoming more important to every aspect of business, including the laboratory. The enabling software technology which will support the increasing demand for data sharing is, of course, database.

Database technology is more than just computer programs used to store and retrieve bits and pieces of data. In the past, computer application systems were written to execute in a more or less serial fashion. At the risk of over-simplifying an extremely complex environment — one program would run which created a data file which would be read by the next program, which produced new data in a file which would be read by the next program, and so on. Each system used a set of data structures which were independent of other systems, and probably different from the structures of any other system.

Even for those systems analysts using commercial database products, system integration was difficult. Database tools of the early- and mid-1980s did not provide an easy way to integrate applications. When a new program needed to interface to an existing database, if the database didn't contain all the required new data fields (which was usually the case), a new database would have to be created containing the new fields and then all the data were copied from the old database.

Because of the difficulty and complexity of integrating computer systems and then maintaining them, large support groups evolved throughout the 1970s and 1980s. Today, a new database technology is offering solutions to the complexity and expense of integrating computer applications. This new technology is the *relational database*. It is important to realize the significance of this technology. In fact, entire corporate MIS strategies are being built around relational database solutions. Development and maintenance costs of integrated computing solutions, using this database technology, will be substantially less than in the past.

How will this new technology accomplish these things? Simply put, the database will become the common thread for all applications. Most importantly, and unlike before, new data types and data fields can be added to the database environment without having to modify any of the existing application programs. Thus, the need for programming staffs will decrease substantially.

How will database technology affect laboratory computing? By providing effective, economically attractive methods for integrating solutions, database technology will result in the continuing use of the departmental minicomputer, throughout the 1990s. Laboratories will continue to be supported with VAX and HP computing capabilities to take advantage of large database applications, and this is where LIMS fits in. Small laboratories will be able to take advantage of PC based LIMS, but medium to large labs will rely on multiuser LIMS.

Summary

With the emergence and collapse of information management methods, tools, and technologies, what can we expect to be using in physical and analytical testing laboratories in the coming years? The departmental multiuser minicomputer will remain a mainstay throughout the 1990s. It will be augmented by better software and networked workstations. The software will include LIMS. LIMS will evolve to run on whatever platforms become popular and will surely take advantage of the graphics capabilities of the networked workstations. Distributed database techniques and artificial intelligence will support LIMS growth and adaptation to the newer and faster computer models which will inevitably be developed. LIMS will take advantage of windows, new application-operating system interactions, and exciting new software features which we can't even begin to imagine. Instruments will become true network devices on our local and wide area networks, and connecting a new instrument will be as simple as plugging in a transceiver cable. The analytical laboratory of the 1990s will be a showcase for new developments from computer and instrument vendors and an exciting place to work. The new technology will totally integrate anything related to information management in the lab.

Upgrading manual methods to computer methods must be a top priority in every laboratory. More than a general commitment to the concept of automation is required. Information management must become part of strategic planning. Short-range laboratory plans (in the 1- to 2-year range) should include the following:

LIMS
A commitment to quality
Travel to conferences showcasing automation and LIMS
Chemical word processing
Statistical process control
Design of experiments
Training lab members in new methods of doing old jobs

Long range plans should include networking and staying current with hardware and software developments.

Chapter 3

Laboratory Automation

A Recollection of Days Gone By

In 1969, a young man employed as a chemist by one of the South's largest coal mining companies was routinely running lab tests on several substrates, including coal and water. The water samples, which were collected from ponds, streams, lakes, and wells near strip mine operations, were being analyzed for mineral content and pH. The number of water samples increased slowly for several months, from an average of 50 to 100 per week. The chemist and his only lab partner were able to accommodate the additional samples without much trouble. Suddenly, without warning, the number of water samples began increasing rapidly. Within 3 months they had increased to over 500 samples per week.

The chemist went to company management with a proposal in his mind and a hand-written contract. Within a month he had resigned his job, opened his own laboratory (with a small bank loan for the needed equipment and supplies), and had a contract for analysis of all the water samples that the coal company generated.

During the first 6 months, while paying off the loan, the chemist's earnings were about the same as when he was with the coal company. Then word of his reasonable price per analysis spread, and soon he was doing business with three coal companies. At the end of 1 year, his income had nearly doubled. However, he was working 7 days per week, 12 hours per day, and still falling behind. It was clear that something had to be done.

His primary objectives became to reduce his work to 50 hours per week and hold his income loss to a minimum. His options were:

1. Reduce number of samples
2. Hire a technician
3. Become more efficient

Option 1 — reduce the number of samples. The chemist calculated that if he reduced the number of samples to a level requiring 50 hours of work per week, his income would drop by approximately $250 per week. One of the problems with this solution was that the number of samples was increasing. His customers were expecting more, not less. The probability was high that his customers would discontinue sending all samples if he asked them to reduce the number. Thus, he might end up losing more than $250 per week.

Option 2 — hire a technician. A technician, working for 40 hours per week, would cost approximately $150 per week. With the help of a technician the chemist felt that he could reduce his workweek to 50 hours and handle the current number of samples.

Option 3 — become more efficient. By adding a calorimeter with an analog strip chart recorder (for coal analyses) and a sample processor which would automatically provide up to 15 aliquots (for water analyses), the chemist could handle the same number of samples and reduce his workweek to 50 hours. The payment on the loan necessary to provide the new equipment would be $50 per week.

The choice was obvious. To accomplish his primary objective of maintaining his income with less personal effort, option 3 was by far the most economically attractive.

This story illustrates the benefit of increased efficiency due to processing more samples in a given time. We may find ourselves in a more complex and scaled up laboratory environment, but we must never lose sight of the fact that productivity can be increased by either adding staff or increasing efficiency, and the latter is almost always preferred.

Automation versus Mechanization

Does the above story illustrate laboratory automation? Upon first consideration, it certainly would seem so; however, Russell Ackoff (6) points that out there is a fundamental difference between automation and mechanization. The concepts of mechanization deal with the replacement of muscle, whereas those of automation deal with the replacement of mind. The use of a machine as a mechanical device to replace human activity is thus not necessarily automation. If the machine does not apply an element of knowledge or decision making, then mechanization, not automation has occurred. So, in light of this clarification, the chemist actually mechanized his lab by adding the sample processor and the recorder equipped calorimeter. Instead of merely recording the combustion temperatures, if the calorimeter had calculated the sample's BTU rating, would this be considered automation? Probably so, although there may be room for arguments.

Some examples may help us better comprehend the difference between mechanization and automation:

1. The early telephone switching systems were mechanized. They used an operator to connect one circuit to another by plugging and unplugging wires, but this required considerably less muscle than twisting the wires together would have needed. At least they were mechanized compared to their immediate successors, the electromechanical switches, which required no muscle. Of course, the new digital switches are required to perform many more automated tasks, such as adaptive routing, billing, and providing call statistics, but when it comes to their primary function — switching circuits — they are no more automated than their electromechanical predecessors.

2. In process control, the recording of temperature values for a process variable was mechanized long ago. Strip chart recorders are still widely used, but they have been replaced in many applications by computers for faster, more accurate, and more responsive monitoring. The simple act of recording a temperature by a machine is not automation. We shift from mechanization to automation when we are able to let the computer decide what should be done about the measurement. If it is in limits, do one thing or possibly nothing. If it is out of limits, do something different, such as notifying an operator or initiating an expert system to make further automated decisions.

3. Chromatographic detection systems became automated when they calculated not only the area, but also the concentration. The replacement of a recorder with an integrator was mechanization. A person was no longer required to measure peaks with a ruler. The addition of a computer to calculate the concentration removed all human effort from the measurement calculation.

4. Is the automobile a mechanized or an automated machine? For the overall machine, the answer has to be that it is mechanized. It certainly removes the muscle component in transporting someone from one place to another, but its use requires more mental power than does walking. The automobile does contain some automated systems which do remove the mental element from driving, such as the automatic choke and cruise control.

What is Laboratory Automation?

Using the distinctions set forth above, we can now say that there is a difference between laboratory automation and laboratory mechanization. Mechanization has existed in the laboratory for a long time. With the advent of Large-Scale Integration (LSI) technology, we now have CPUs in many of lab instruments, allowing us to classify them as automated.

The drive behind laboratory automation is always, without exception, enhanced productivity. Laboratory automation systems have increased productivity by providing benefits such as the following: (1) calculation and transcription errors associated with copying data values from one piece of paper to another are significantly reduced, (2) records of who did what, how and when it was done, and any subsequent modifications are maintained automatically, [and] (3) "the working day can be extended from 8 to 18 hours without multiple shifts or additional staff" (36). Of course, we could accomplish all these things with manual methods if we hired enough personnel, but how much would it cost?

The necessity for laboratory automation has engendered LIMS technology. Before we can derive the exact relationship between LIMS and laboratory automation, it is necessary to break laboratory automation down into its components. The two primary components are automated laboratory instrumentation and automated laboratory information management. Both offer tremendous economic benefits (2,3) and they go hand-in-hand. In fact, the employment of automated instrumentation increases the number of samples and the amount of sample data, quickly rendering manual information management methods inadequate. As laboratories come to use more and more automated instrumentation, we have no choice but to look for automated methods of information management. Figure 3-1 depicts laboratory automation as an interwoven mesh of its two primary components. In the following sections, we further separate this mesh into its subgroups and individual subcomponents.

Automated Laboratory Instrumentation

The use of automated instrumentation means that we have removed both the muscle and mind components in obtaining analytical results. Automated instruments automate the processes of data production. More samples can be run in a given amount of time using such instruments. The data produced tend to yield greater precision and more precise methods or measurements, and fewer samples are required to obtain desired confidence levels.

Figure 3-2 shows that automated laboratory instrumentation has two major components — data acquisition and instrument management.

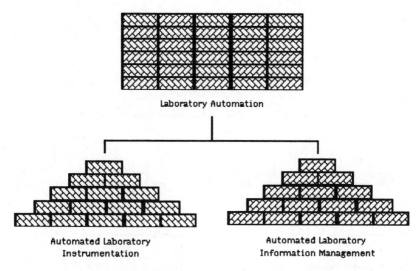

Figure 3-1. Laboratory automation — composed of two major components.

These concepts define how to connect computers and robots to instruments, how to control instrument operation, and how to transfer measurement data to a computer. In the recent past, data acquisition techniques were not simple and instrument management was done by manual methods. The following sections examine these two important aspects of automated laboratory instrumentation.

Data Acquisition.   Humans can acquire data by manually writing test results on a worksheet or in a notebook; however, manual methods are usually not what is meant by the term *data acquisition*. Instead, this term refers to the automatic collection of raw data, usually by a computer. Computer collection points for data, whether in the instrument itself, in a local PC or lab computer, or on a superminicomputer host, should be considered part of the data acquisition system. Robotic sample handling systems which present samples to the instrument should be considered part of data acquisition when their actions are controlled by the computer system. The storage of the raw data is the logical end of data acquisition.

Figure 3-3 describes the components of automated laboratory instrumentation and illustrates some of the major facets of data acquisition. Data acquisition systems have shown strong progress over the last 10-15 years. In the early 1970s, computers with complicated A/D modules were required for data acquisition. Now the minimum we expect on a laboratory instrument is a computer connection, and most are computer controlled with their own built-in CPUs. But although we have come a

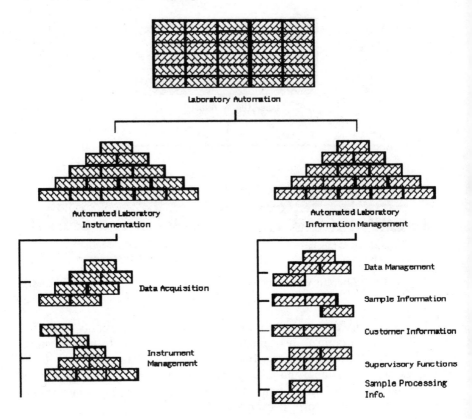

Figure 3-2. Laboratory automation — major components and subcomponents.

long way, instrument-computer interfaces are by no means standard. We have been warned many times about the "standard" RS-232 interface, which is really nonstandard. And even when the communications link does work, that is just the beginning (40,41). Some custom programming is usually required to interface an instrument to a computer because the report and data output formats are all different. There are no standards. For some this programming is easy, but for others it is a show stopper.

Some writers have suggested that "any laboratory instrument that has an electrical interface capable of transmitting result data to an external device, be it a printer or a computer, may be interfaced to a LIMS computer system" (39). Others have stated that "complex custom software must often be developed for each instrument interfaced" (40). Both of these observations are true. The indeterminate variable is the phrase *complex custom*. A complex problem to some may be basic to others. At this point, it is important to note that instrument interfacing is possible.

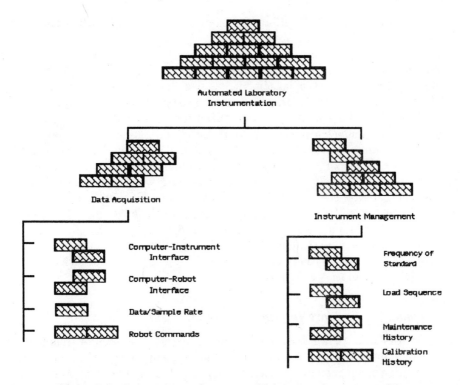

Figure 3-3. Components of automated laboratory instrumentation.

(Customization and tailoring of LIMS are briefly examined in Chapter 4 and dealt with in detail in Chapter 12. Data acquisition systems and instrument management systems are discussed in Chapter 7.)

Enabling data acquisition is easier for some instruments than for others. By the same token, its easier to enable data acquisition for some commercial LIMS packages than for others. As we will describe in Chapter 12, there is strong evidence that the LIMS vendors are attempting to make the data acquisition features of their products very flexible and usable. No one doubts that data acquisition is a focal point of laboratory automation. It is a major feature of some commercial LIMS products, and it can be built into others. The next few years will be filled with breakthroughs in the area of the LIMS-data acquisition interface. Software standards will be developed to make it easier to connect instruments to computers and to acquire data via the LIMS.

The future of laboratory data acquisition is exciting. Laboratory computing and instrument vendors will adhere to standards as they are adopted. Computers and instruments of all brands and models will be plug compatible. When will it happen? Not immediately. As we take each step toward high level standardization, connectivity will become easier and less expensive.

Instrument Management.   Figure 3-3 illustrates some of the major components of instrument management. As we can see, this function is related to the use and maintenance of an instrument. Although systems for controlling instruments have been used for a long time, the concept of instrument management goes beyond merely operating the instrument to analyze samples. Having the instrument run a standard sample at a given interval is part of instrument management, as is having the instrument automatically rerun a standard sample when a certain result limit range is exceeded. Comparison of test results by running the same sample on more than one instrument can provide calibration for the instrument(s). Making this comparison at a given interval is part of instrument management. Calibration and maintenance histories are becoming more important as labs comply with GLP guidelines and strive for high-quality output.

Automated Laboratory Information Management

Laboratory information has many components, as described in Chapter 2. Data management is one of the five primary components of laboratory information management, as seen in Figure 3-2. The others are sample information, customer information, supervisory functions, and sample processing information. Some of the information types which make up these primary components are illustrated in Figure 3-4. The application of automated computer processes to the use of these types of laboratory information is what we term *automated laboratory information management*.

There is a difference between computerized information management and automated information management. Computerized information management should be regarded as merely more efficient, extended manual methods. Information management is not automated just because it is computerized. Certainly, getting data into the database is the first step in automated information management, but it is what we do with the data after computerizing them that determines their maximum benefit potential. Data management systems have been used to automate data collection — getting the data into the database. These systems offer some automated features, such as automatic archival and report generation.

Automated methods of processing sample information are provided in automated laboratory information management. Logging of samples into and out of the lab, automatic report generation upon review of the test results, and automatic production of work lists are examples of sample

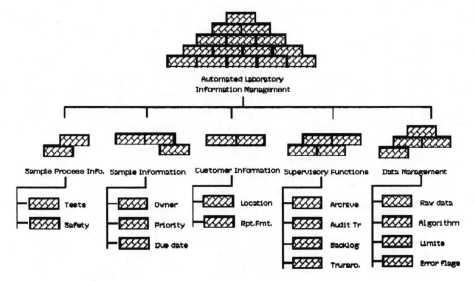

Figure 3-4. Components of automated laboratory information management.

information processing which can be automated. Customer information items, such as report destination, no longer need to be dealt with by the analyst because they are taken care of by the system.

Automated laboratory information management supervisory functions offer benefits which may seem intangible at first, but upon further examination, can clearly add to productivity. For example, a function of most current LIMS is the *backlog*. What most systems actually have are manual *backlog reporting mechanisms*, which can produce sample backlog reports on command or even automatically at a certain time each day. Imagine taking this function a step further and implementing an automated *backlog management system* (BMS).

Our BMS could be set up with limits on both high and low sides. If the backlog fell lower than expected, a flag would be raised which might indicate one of the following:

A new operator or mailperson is taking samples to the wrong laboratory.
Your customer has gone out of business.
Your efficiency has increased to the point where you can reduce the staff.

A high flag might indicate one of the following:

An instrument has failed.
Training is needed.

The number of samples has increased.
Additional staff or instruments are needed.

Whether a high or low limit was reached, any of these situations would require attention - and the sooner the better. You might suppose that the operator responsible for the particular analysis would go to the lab manager with the backlog problem, but that is not necessarily true. Our BMS could contain an expert system which, through database and operator inquiries, would suggest possible actions to assist the operator in assigning a probable cause.

The management of sample backlog information provides a key measure related to resource allocation. Manual methods to report and plot backlogs, look for backlog trends, and flag and find causes for upsets would require so much time that, more often than not, they would be neglected. The system that automatically prints or plots backlog reports is very close to what we could consider an automated system but it does not force any action when a limit is exceeded. A fully automated system will force an action, even if the action is manual, such as simply acknowledging the error flag.

Sample processing information, such as which tests are required for which sample, no longer have to be manually read from a form accompanying the samples. Samples are automatically scheduled for the proper tests. Even reruns are scheduled automatically.

Until recently, manual and semiautomated computer methods were sufficient to handle the amounts of information generated by lab analysts. However, it must be realized that many information management functions, which seemed less important than data generation in the past, have been neglected. Today, when we are able to process more and more samples via automated methods and instruments, we are increasing the sample/analyst ratio. The choice is clear: Either hire enough clerks to manage the information or automate information management. The latter is the obvious choice.

Relationship Between Laboratory Automation and LIMS

As stated above, until recently analysts were able to manage much of the information flowing through physical and analytical testing laboratories. A combination of manual and computer assisted manual methods were adequate for most lab requirements. Today, new laboratory instrumentation, robotics, and other automation techniques produce more information than our analysts can handle. In the past, instrument speed or calculations limited turnaround time; now there are many other reasons. The keying of sample information and subsequent test results into computer systems is one such information bottleneck.

Dealing with more and more of the same information which was once handled manually is not the complete problem. Laboratory personnel must also manage types of information which had low priority in the past but are now becoming more important, such as audit trails and instrument calibration histories. The commitment to quality performance and the need for compliance with federal regulations are changing the way we think about these types of information.

A LIMS, properly implemented, can help alleviate information bottlenecks. In fact, recognition of the need to manage all types of laboratory information is the driving force behind the development of the LIMS application technology. As we saw above, a BMS is an example of automated laboratory information management. It can easily be built within a LIMS. A LIMS thus provides the "culture" for growing automated laboratory information management, which is one-half of laboratory automation. LIMS functions provide a "backbone" on which to build laboratory automation. The LIMS backbone concept is also valid for the other half of laboratory automation - automated instrumentation. Projects involving computerized acquisition of data from instruments can have a common data repository — the LIMS database. What better storage place could there be? Programs controlling data acquisition either come with LIMS packages or can be built as part of LIMS functions.

Summary

We have looked at laboratory automation as a means of achieving enhanced efficiency. New generations of laboratory instruments and new computer methods to automate old instruments are allowing us to process more samples with fewer personnel. Laboratory robots work three shifts a day turning out data and more data. In order to prevent a productivity bottleneck, we must computerize and automate data management and associated information management processes. The integration of collecting, processing, and communicating all laboratory information is the essence of the new technology. It will encompass all aspects of lab processes and procedures.

The implementation of a LIMS provides instant computerization of laboratory data and other information. The LIMS also provides the backbone on which to build the necessary automated instrumentation and automated information management processes, to carry us through the 1990s. There is no plateau of laboratory efficiency toward which we should work. We will continuously be faced with reasons for enhancing performance — this is the nature of today's competitive world.

Section Two

LIMS Functions

Chapter 4

Introduction to Laboratory
Information Management Systems

To this point, we have examined many of the concepts and practices related to the use of computers in analytical laboratories. We have stated that a LIMS provides the information management tools that lab analysts require to manage the tremendous amount of information which they are required to handle. In Chapter 5 we begin looking in detail at LIMS functions — what they do, how they work, and how the different commercial packages implement the various functions. This in-depth look at individual LIMS functions will be better understood if we first review all the functions and the sequence in which we expect them to be used.

Many organizations are either considering LIMS or are using it already. This chapter begins by examining the ways in which these organizations first became familiar with the LIMS concept. A general overview of the important functions and features of the LIMS environment is then presented. We also begin a comparison of the following commercial LIMS packages:

1. Axiom Systems, Inc., "VM LIMS"
2. Beckman Instruments, Inc., "CALS Lab Manager"
3. Digital Equipment Corp., "LIMS/SM"
4. Hewlett-Packard Company, "LABSAM"
5. Perkin Elmer Nelson Systems, Inc., "RLAB"
6. Perkin Elmer Nelson Systems, Inc., "LIMS 2000"
7. Perkin Elmer Nelson Systems, Inc., "ACCESS*LIMS"
8. Varian, "LIMS/DM"
9. VG Laboratory Systems Limited, "Sample Manager"

The purpose of the comparisons throughout is mainly to point out similarities between LIMS packages and to highlight unique features. By looking at these differences and similarities, we can better understand the objectives of particular functions and features. There is no intention of suggesting that any LIMS is in any way better than another. Every laboratory operates differently because of the variations among lab operators, analysts, and managers. Different instrument interface requirements, varying numbers of samples, computer hardware selection, and many other determinants will influence which LIMS is best suited for a particular laboratory or group of laboratories. The decision as to which LIMS is best is left up to those who may need to make that decision. The purpose of these comparisons is to help understand LIMS. Product evaluations must be done carefully and extensively with hands on testing, as described in Chapter 11.

As noted in Chapter 1, there are approximately 20 commercial LIMS available. The ones selected here for comparison include some of the more mature products, as well as certain newer ones. With any computer software, maturity demands respect; and LIMS is no exception. Software that doesn't improve with time will die. When a new software product is introduced, there is a good chance that it will be better in many ways than many of its competitors. New and better features offered for a lower price will always gain attention in the marketplace. This is the essence of free enterprise and the basis for growth in any industry, including computer software. We should never exclude a software product from evaluation just because it or its company is new. But maturity, respect, and solidness of the vendor organization should weigh very heavily in any product evaluation. Software companies come and go every day.

LIMS Champion

At most organizations either considering a LIMS installation or with a LIMS already in place, there is a person responsible for developing the initial interest in LIMS. This person, after gaining initial interest, either becomes the LIMS champion or finds another person or group to further develop enthusiasm for the LIMS project. This person is employed by the lab as either a scientist or a computer support worker. Many scientists generate the initial interest in LIMS within a testing facility. The scientist's first contact with a LIMS may come from reading about it in the technical literature, from an acquaintance with another firm using LIMS, from a vendor contact, from a vendor user group meeting, or from a consultant. Other possible sources of initial contact are scientific conferences such as the Pittsburgh Conference, the Association of Official Analytical Chemists (AOAC) Conference, the Scientific Computing and Automation Conference, or from the American Chemical Society (ACS). At these conferences, much space and effort are being dedicated to LIMS demonstrations and technical sessions by various LIMS vendors and LIMS users.

Another source of LIMS information for scientists has been the International LIMS Meetings, presented by the Laboratory Information Management Systems Institute, Inc. These conferences are dedicated to LIMS information sharing. Many case studies are presented by users who have gained experience with LIMS. Vendors participate mainly by helping with the organization and staging of the meeting and with poster session demonstrations.

As stated above, the LIMS champion may belong to a computer support group within a laboratory or group of laboratories. Some laboratories have computer application support as a laboratory function. The degree of support will vary, depending on laboratory size, from a part-time use of one person to a group or even a whole organization. The possible sources of available information which may pique the interest of the computer support person about LIMS are, of course, the same as for the scientist.

Similarity of Commercially Available LIMS

Computers are machines which perform certain functions better than humans. Computer programs translate the steps of a particular function into a code that is understood by the computer. We can thus think of computer programs as the interface between human methods and computer methods. Software development, in many cases, is the extension of human experience to computer methods. Developers of software draw on their own experience, or that of their clients, to produce computer programs which emulate human behavior or thinking.

In a laboratory environment where samples are processed, a set of practices or procedures is used to generate the samples and deliver them to the lab. Other procedures or methods are used to process the samples and return the test results. Although laboratories and samples differ greatly, there is a similarity in the practices, procedures, and methods associated with sample processing. LIMS software translates these practices, procedures, and methods into computer methods.

As we might expect, the similarity of sample processing practices, procedures, and methods is responsible for the similarity between commercially available LIMS packages. LIMS software developers have extended a set of similar manual methods to a set of similar computer methods. This is not to say that all LIMS packages are alike, only that many of them have similar functionality and structure.

The LIMS Environment

Status

When samples come into a testing laboratory, they may be assigned to an analyst or to a particular test. They may be placed on a work list or routed to a particular instrument. Regardless of how a sample is processed, its status will undergo a series of changes during its stay in the testing laboratory. A sample will have a different status while it is being tested than it does at other times. When all required tests are completed, the status will change again. Thus, the status of a sample which is processed in an analytical lab will change several times between its creation and the archiving of its test results.

Many sample submitters have one attribute in common: From time to time, they all want test results more quickly than the testing lab can provide them. As a result, they regularly call the lab to inquire about the status of a particular sample or group of samples. The lab analyst must interrupt the work that she or he is currently doing to check on the sample(s). This delays not only the work in progress but all other work in the queue. It may take only a minute or two to satisfy the request, but if it happens 10 times per day, that's 1.66 hours per week. What is the consequence of delaying results for all the lab's samples? Although it's hard quantify this type of loss, it is probably significant.

Most LIMS allow the sample submitter to obtain the status of sample(s) without assistance from the lab analyst. A LIMS function, sometimes called *sample progress*, can be run from the submitter's own terminal at any time. The sample progress function displays the status of the sample, along with any test results which have already been entered by the testing lab. Thus, with the use of the sample status and the sample progress function, LIMS puts an information management tool in the hands of the user. Instant access to sample status and test results is provided, which without LIMS would require a phone call or two.

As we review the various LIMS functions, we will find many opportunities for improving lab operations. We will examine the sample progress utility and others in more detail and give examples in Chapter 10.

Appendix A-1 presents an excerpt from Varian Associates' *LIMS/DM User's Manual*. The sections titled "The Sample States" and "The Test States" are taken from the chapter, "System Description." They are presented here because they provide an excellent description of status. We note also that a sample isn't the only LIMS object to which a status is assigned. Tests also carry a status indicator. Reviewing these sections gives us an appreciation of the intricacies involved in LIMS sample management. It also provides a fairly in-depth look at sample flow within a LIMS.

Referencing these sections in this introductory chapter may be like learning how to swim by jumping into 10-feet-deep water, but they give us a quick look at many LIMS functions. Many of these functions operate by managing sample and test statuses. For example, the LIMS backlog function operates by searching the database for samples which have a status that indicates that they are not complete. The purpose of approving a sample's test results, as far as LIMS itself is concerned, is to change the sample status from "complete" to "approved." Thus, the internal operation of a LIMS, from data entry to database searching, is based on one form or another of a status condition or change.

LIMS Functions

The following is a description of LIMS functions which we would expect to find in any LIMS package. Terminology may differ among packages, but the purposes are the same. These descriptions are simplified and abbreviated, but taken collectively, they present an overview of LIMS operation. Many of these functions are described in detail in later chapters. We will also examine how the various functions alter the status of a sample.

Sample Collection.   There are as many different means of sample generation as there are types of samples. Samples can originate from rivers, reactions, process streams, human or nonhuman specimens, pieces of fabric, distillation columns, and so on. Often a reaction will be conducted on the bench top for the sole purpose of producing a sample or samples for chemical or physical analysis. But regardless of the origin, sample collection always goes hand-in-hand with sample generation. In fact, a sample does not exist until it is either collected or ready to be collected.

Sample collection usually involves transfer or placement of the sample into a container such as a small vial, bottle, or envelope. On this container will be placed the sample ID. From this point on, the sample ID will be the sample owner's primary, if not only, reference between sample generation and test results.

Samples which are collected on a schedule can be referred to as *routine samples*. Several LIMS functions offer assistance in handling these samples. For example, (beg-itl)Collection Lists(end-itl) can be generated which provide operators with the information necessary to collect routine samples, such as the sample origin, what time to collect, sample IDs, and what tests will be required.

Sample LOGIN.   Physical and analytical testing laboratories are in business to process samples. Any system, whether electronic or manual, which is used to manage samples must be provided with a certain amount of information about each sample. Sample LOGIN is the LIMS function that provides most or all of the relevant sample information to the system. LOGIN is performed either by the person generating (or collecting) the sample, who is referred to as the *sample submitter*, or by testing lab personnel. Samples are usually logged in before the desired tests are performed. The status of a sample immediately after LOGIN is "logged in". The above mentioned Collection Lists are usually generated in association with sample LOGIN.

The sample LOGIN function requires the sample submitter to enter certain information. Other information is optional. The only information which the LIMS actually has to have to process the sample further is the sample ID and a list of what tests are to be performed; however, the testing lab may require other information such as the charge number and safety information, before a sample can be processed. A fully functional LIMS allows the testing lab to specify which information is required and which is optional.

Sample RECEIVE.   This consists of acknowledgment by testing personnel that a sample has been received in the testing laboratory. Until the sample is received, the lab has no responsibility for it. Some labs, of course, create their own samples. These labs would not benefit from using a RECEIVE function. The sample RECEIVE function changes the status of the sample from "logged" in to "received" or "in lab".

Worksheets and Worklists.   These are lists of samples which have been submitted for testing. They can be generated and sorted in various orders, such as by employee, priority, date due, and test code. Worksheet or worklist generation is done by testing lab personnel, sometimes in conjunction with the RECEIVE step. Some LIMS packages use these lists of samples as an integral part of sample processing. For others, they are optional. In either case, worksheets and worklists are merely information management tools for use by the lab analyst in scheduling samples, tests, or instruments.

Results Entry.   After completion of a test, the results must be entered into the LIMS, usually by one of two methods:

1. Manual results entry — test results are entered from the keyboard.
2. Automatic results entry — test results are transferred from the instrument via an instrument-to-computer connection and automatically entered into the database.

Inclusion of automatic results entry into a LIMS is the single best method to increase productivity in the laboratory and to reduce data entry errors. Some LIMS packages come with automatic results entry built in. Others provide it as an option. And for still other LIMS, automatic results entry is made possible by providing access to user-written code. The ability to provide or accommodate automatic results entry is one of the two most important features of a LIMS.

When the first test result for a sample is entered, the sample's status changes from "in lab" to "under test". When all the results have been entered, the status changes to "complete."

Results Verification. All test results (or interpretations) produced in a testing laboratory should be reviewed and approved before being issued. The review may be performed by the analyst who produced the result(s), another lab member, or the lab manager. Regardless of who is authorized to review and approve results, most LIMS generally provide means to ensure adequate control over data integrity. Some LIMS may require multiple approvals, i.e., the approval of the analyst and the lab manager may be required before a test result can be reported to the sample submitter. In this situation, only the lab manager is allowed to use the "final review" function.

If the reviewer approves the result, the sample status changes from "complete" to "reviewed and approved." If the reviewer does not approve the result, the status changes to "reviewed and disapproved." When a result is not approved, the LIMS can be instructed to request a retest of the analysis.

Reporting Results. As soon as the status of a sample becomes reviewed and approved, the test results can be reported. In many cases, the results will be reported to the sample submitter. In other cases, there may be one particular operator, chemist, or engineer who processes results from several submitters. Most LIMS provide for electronic results reporting, a major step toward paperless systems. Some LIMS allow selection of the report destination, such as the submitter's electronic mailbox, an electronic spreadsheet, or a file in the submitter's personal directory.

The above functions are not the only ones we would expect to find in a LIMS. They are simply the basic functions necessary to process a sample, which is certainly not the highest function of a LIMS. Other higher-level functions that provide information management tools were not listed, but are considered in later chapters.

Sequencing of LIMS Standard Functions

In the above sections, we looked at a collection of procedures, or functions, ranging from sample generation and collection to test results reporting. We can summarize these functions to a sequence which can be viewed as an expected or normal sample processing sequence:

1. Sample collection (with optional Collection List generation)
2. Sample LOGIN
3. Sample RECEIVE
4. Optional worksheet generation
5. Results entry
6. Results verification
7. Results Reporting

Because most LIMS provide these functions, we can consider them as basic or even standard. We see these functions in Appendixes A-2, A-3, A-4, and A-5, which present sample processing flowcharts of some of the popular commercial LIMS packages. These examples also display some differences in nomenclature, as well as certain steps unique to one package. Only one of the flow examples shows *Print Labels*, which are, of course, barcode labels. But this example isn't the only one of this group to use barcode labels. Thus, these flowcharts were not designed by the vendors to illustrate all the products' functions. There are some similarities. They each start with logging in samples, and all produce reports somewhere near the end.

Core Functions

As indicated above, certain functions are included in almost all LIMS packages. This group of functions is called the *standard functions*. Finding such similarity among packages is not surprising because they are all designed to solve the same problems. Thus, we would expect all LIMS packages to be similar in some regards. Some very important questions have arisen concerning these similarities. Which functions should we always expect to find in any package which is advertised as a LIMS? Should a software package contain a certain set of core functions before it can be advertised as a LIMS? Most LIMS vendors agree that it should. But as we might foresee, there will be much discussion of this topic. The ASTM E31.4 committee on LIMS has become the forum for these discussions. This committee, which is composed of LIMS vendors, as well as chemical and pharmaceutical industry representatives, has the goal of defining the core LIMS functions. (Other significant projects of the committee which are in dire need of standards are laboratory communications and terminology.)

Differences Among LIMS

We have noted that the similarity among commercial LIMS packages is to be expected. So, if many LIMS packages are similar and offer the same standard functions, then how do they differ? Some of the primary differences lie in how the following are applied to all LIMS functions:

Database technology   Statistical analysis
Graphics   Customization
Communications   Instrumentation interfacing
Tailorability   Security
Integration with other systems

None of the above are trivial considerations. Their relative importance varies among LIMS installations. Customization, tailorability, and database technology are perhaps the most important factors. Good customization and tailoring techniques can make up for shortcomings in other areas. The database design, regardless of the database type or organization, must be very responsive (fast) and provide flexible, easy access to the data. We will now briefly examine database technology, customization, and tailorability, not to point out specific differences between LIMS packages, but to stress their importance.

Database Technology

A LIMS is a database application. The entire system is built around a database. The database is the heart of the system, and the database input/output (I/O) is its lifeblood. The speed of database operations determines the responsiveness of the system. Of course, hardware horsepower has a strong effect on responsiveness but, relatively speaking, faster database I/O means a faster LIMS.

Database technology has advanced significantly in the past 5-10 years. Relational database technology has become the most heavily advertised and most popular form in the past 5 years. As stated in Chapter 2, this technology will have a major impact on computing in the coming years. By the year 2000, it is likely that all LIMS will be using a relational database or whatever new technology evolves to replace it.

Today, some LIMS use a hierarchical database design, some use a CODASYL (ANSI Conference On DAta SYstems Languages) database, and some use a relational database. Some advertise their database structure as a strong feature, and others don't mention it at all. Some vendors have built their LIMS on a commercial database product, and some have designed their own database. Figure 4-1 shows which of our comparison products have which type of database.

What are the differences between relational and hierarchical databases? Which is best for a LIMS? "Laboratory data are most naturally expressed as a hierarchical construct consisting of sample header information, test header information, and test results" (43). This statement certainly seems to answer the question of which database type is best. Of course, it was made by the LIMS product line manager of a vendor with a hierarchical database product. Those with relational database LIMS packages probably feel the same about their product.

What are the most important features of the database that affect its performance? Some of them are size, speed, ease of use, security, auditing, shadowing (or mirroring), backup, and failure protection. Some features, such as speed and ease of use, are more important to the end user, while others such as failure protection and backup, are more important to support personnel. The current belief in the computer industry is that while relational database technology may be slower, it is easier to search, program, and set up.

As we describe in Chapter 11, ad hoc database searching is a very powerful feature of a LIMS application. It allows the LIMS user to rapidly devise search strategies for selecting data relationships without the need for complicated database programming. Also associated with relational databases is the use of SQL, the ANSI standard language for relational databases. SQL, also referred to as IBM's *structured query language* (20,44), has a high degree of database searching flexibility. Some LIMS are beginning to combine relational database technology

	AXIOM	B EC CA KL MS A N	L I DM ES C/ S M	L A HB PS A M	N ER PLL ESA OB N	2 P0 E0 0	NA EC PLC ESE OS NS	V L A I RM I S A / ND M	M A VN GA G E R
Hierarchical database				X					
Relational database	X				X	X	X		X
CODASYL database			X					X	
Uses proprietary database		X		X					X

Figure 4-1. LIMS comparison — database related.

and SQL search mechanisms to provide ad hoc search capability. If ad hoc searching is needed to fulfill the search requirements for some LIMS users, then a LIMS with a relational database and SQL may be desirable.

How many of us with a LIMS in place know what kind of database it uses? How many of us care as long as the database is fast, easy to maintain, and provides all the search capability we need? So, even though the difference in database technology may be one of the significant differences between LIMS products, the type of database used is unimportant as long as it is responsive to the needs of its users and provides an avenue for future growth.

Customization and Tailorability

Customization and tailorability are both considered important distinctions between different LIMS packages. Both are advertised by various vendors. Although related, they have different meanings in terms of LIMS software. They are related in that both may change the appearance of the LIMS to the user. They differ in the degree of change. Tailoring may involve changing menus or phrases on display screens, help text, error messages, and report formats. Customization may involve adding all new functions, interfacing new and different instruments, and interfacing to other software systems, such as accounting and billing.

The standard LIMS functions are the building blocks for developing and customizing systems in any laboratory. The degree of customization needed in a particular laboratory depends on the size and complexity of the LIMS being implemented. More test methods mean that more types of instrumentation must be interfaced. More users mean more requests for customizations. One LIMS package may be a turnkey system for one laboratory, while only providing a starting point for others. Regardless of what features users are looking for in a LIMS, or even if they simply want the LIMS with the most and best features, it is necessary to evaluate LIMS with a "hidden" understanding. A LIMS which is advertised to solve all problems may provide basis for doing so but may also require a lot of work.

There is another group of LIMS functions which we will call the LIMS supervisory functions. Although they can easily be standard functions for any LIMS package, they were not so listed above because they are not required to process a sample. They are discussed in Chapter 10.

Summary

We have listed a sequence of functions associated with sample processing. Because they are provided by most commercially available LIMS packages, we have termed them the standard LIMS functions.

These standard functions appear to provide nothing new. This sequence has been followed in laboratories for years, generally with the use of manual and paper methods; however, as noted above, this is to be expected. Today's LIMS packages are applying computer technology to existing laboratory methods and procedures. We have increased laboratory efficiency and output quality by making existing methods more responsive to customers' needs. Thus, the new technology is evolving. As we find new ways to incorporate computer and information management technologies into lab processes, we further the new technology's development. And lab customers will benefit directly.

The difference between tailoring and customizing was defined as mainly one of degree. A LIMS may offer extensive tailorability, but if it cannot be customized to interface to the lab's instrumentation, it might not improve efficiency. The degree of customization required for a LIMS to provide an efficiency improvement path for the future, is one of the most important considerations when evaluating LIMS packages. Some customization will most likely be required; thus, ease of customization may be the most important feature. We must make sure that we can change the LIMS as needed. Users, after a few months of getting used to the system, will keep us busy with many useful suggestions for improvement.

Chapter 5

Sample LOGIN and Collection Lists

Sample LOGIN

As described in Chapter 2, the amount of sample information managed by a LIMS is extensive. In Chapter 4 we saw that sample LOGIN is typically considered the first step in the routine use of a LIMS. Sample LOGIN is the function performed to enter most or all of the relevant information about a sample into the system and usually involves filling out a form on the terminal screen. As described below, it can be done either before or after the sample has been generated and either before or after the sample has been taken to the laboratory for testing.

In some laboratory environments the sample creator logs her or his own samples into the LIMS. This person could be a scientist in a research laboratory or a plant operator sampling a production run. In other environments, the submitter merely takes samples to the testing lab, where they are logged into the LIMS by lab personnel. In either case, the information entered for sample LOGIN is the same. This information may include the following:

A sample ID	Origin, originator, or owner
Sample type	Date drawn
Date due	Required tests
Aliquot IDs	Test limits
Comments	Report format
Safety factors	Report destination
Charge number	Retain data date

There are two main methods, or sequences, for logging in samples:

1. Prelogging — LOGIN is done before the required tests are performed.
2. Postlogging — LOGIN is done after the required tests are performed.

Prelogged Samples

Most of the time, sample LOGIN is done prior to sample testing. Thus, we should think of the position of sample LOGIN in the following sequence as the norm:

sample generation → sample LOGIN → analysis → results report

This sequence is certainly followed when samples are being generated on a nonroutine and/or low volume basis. But even for routine, high volume testing, this sequence is preferred by most laboratories. Generally, most LIMS packages are designed to operate using this sequence. In most instances, information entered during sample LOGIN is needed before the test can be performed. Sample type and safety information must be known before the test is performed. Information entered during sample LOGIN is also used to obtain sample counts for each requested test method. This information is used to schedule the lab's operation related to analysts and instruments.

Batch LOGIN.   Some commercially available LIMS packages provide an automatic method for prelogging samples, which is an important and very useful feature. Production, control, or routine samples can be logged automatically by the system with no human intervention, and is sometimes referred to as *batch LOGIN*. These samples are processed in the following sequence:

sample LOGIN → sample generation → analysis → results report

For example, an operator might be required to draw a sample from each of 10 process streams every hour. All samples for the operator's shift could be prelogged at one sitting. The samples could even be prelogged automatically by the system days in advance. Many times, "prelogged samples" actually means samples that are logged into the LIMS before they are created. At other times, these samples are logged in before testing is completed.

Postlogged Samples

It is sometimes necessary to analyze samples before logging them into a LIMS. Thus, all sample data including the typical LOGIN information as well as the test results, must be presented to the LIMS at the same time. Some commercially available LIMS packages have this feature. It can be referred to as LOGIN-WITH-RESULTS. The processing sequence would then be:

sample generation → analysis → sample LOGIN → results report

This situation can be called *postanalysis LOGIN*. Some example cases for postanalysis LOGIN are as follows:

1. A remote or isolated computer, or any laboratory without a dedicated computer link may collect sample information and test results to be batched into the LIMS database, perhaps at some regular interval or off hours. In this case, the primary function of the LIMS is data archival, and it may produce summary reports of data collected over some time period.
2. As mentioned in Chapter Two, some laboratories generate their own samples and use the test results internally. If a data management system requires input of a sample ID, it would be redundant to reenter the ID into the LIMS. The sample ID and the corresponding test results could be transferred to the LIMS in a postanalysis sequence. For example, a laboratory generates samples which are to be analyzed on its own gas chromatograph (GC). A data system connected to the GC instrument prompts the analyst for a sample ID before processing. The data system then collects the raw data and analyzes the chromatogram. The sample ID, retention times, peak areas, and component concentrations are then moved to the LIMS. A sample LOGIN-WITH-RESULTS is performed. The data is captured for eternity and made available to the LIMS processes and users.

Figure 5-1 lists the sample LOGIN options offered by our comparison LIMS products. Examples of sample LOGIN screens are as follows:

1. Figure 5-2 — Varian LIMS/DM
2. Figure 5-3 — DEC LIMS/SM
3. Figure 5-4 — PE-Nelson RLAB II
4. Figure 5-5 — AXIOM VM LIMS
5. Figure 5-6 — PE LIMS 2000

As expected, there is a great deal of similarity among the forms. Some look simpler than others at first glance, but may actually require filling out more screens to complete the LOGIN function. Basically, however, they are all the same.

| | B EC CA KL MS A N | L I DM ES C/ S M | L A HB PS A M | N ER PLL ESA OB N | 2 P0 E0 0 | NA EC PLC ESE OS NS | VL A I RM I S A/ ND M | SM SA VMN GPA LG EE R |
	A X I O M								
Sample LOGIN by sample	X	X	X	X	X	X	X	X	X
Prelog samples (batch LOGIN)	X	X	X	X	X	X	X		X
Default Test Code	X	X	X	X	X	X		X	X

Figure 5-1. LIMS comparison — sample LOGIN related.

Required Tests and Default Test Codes

During the LOGIN process, the sample submitter must indicate what analytical/physical test or group of tests is to be performed on the sample. In Figure 5-2 "ASH" is the specified test in the "Method ID field." In Figure 5-3, the desired tests are entered into the "Test Codes" fields. In Figures 5-4, 5-5, and 5-6, there are no fields for entering the desired

```
┌─────────────┐   LIMS/DM                                              Function
│ v a r i a n │   LOGIN SAMPLE
└─────────────┘                              ──────────────── 29-JUL-86 / 06:34 PM
                              Sample ID:       86072900132
External ID: RAWCOAL          Sample Name:     COAL           Client ID: C.R.A.
Due Date:      4-Aug-1986     Sample Type:     RAW            In Lab:   Y
Priority:    5                Sample Source:   BIN #5         Login By: LIMSDM

Sample Description: Raw coal from feeder bin #5, 7/29/86 - 1800 hrs

Precaution Note:    none
Storage Note:       Retain shed
Disposal Note:      Retain till further notice per RDF.

           Ali    Method ID - Section;Version  R  Worklist
            1     ASH         - SAMPLE      ;2   1 ELEMENTALS
                              -             ;
                              -             ;
                              -             ;
                              -             ;

    F1      F2       F3      F4      F5      F6      F7      F8      F9
  LOGIN   COPY     CLEAR
Logged 1 of 1
```

Figure 5-2. Varian LIMS/DM sample LOGIN screen. (Varian Associates. 1986. *Varian Laboratory Data Management User's Manual.* Varian LIMS/DM Version 1.7.1. Walnut Creek, Calif. pp. 5–7)

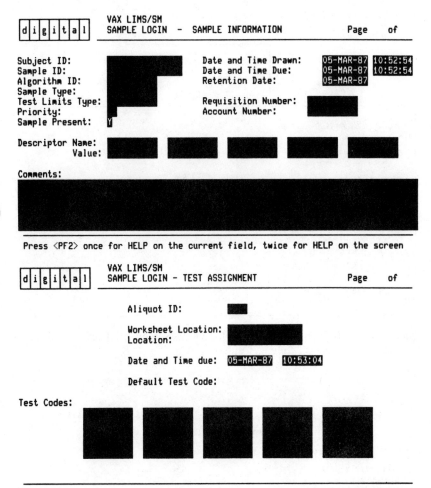

Figure 5-3. DEC LIMS/SM sample LOGIN screen page 1 at top, page 2 at bottom. Digital Equipment Corporation. 1987. *VAX LIMS/SM Planning Workbook*. Maynard, Mass. pp. A-100, A-104)

tests. Instead we see "SAMPLE TYPE," "TYPE OF SAMPLE," and "PROJECT CODE," respectively. These fields are related to the desired tests by a convention known as default test codes. For example, in Figure 5-6, "CRUDE" was entered as the PROJECT CODE. In the lower part of the figure, which is actually page 2 of the Sample LOGIN function, the test codes "RESID," "FLASH," "VISC," "SULFR," and "D2887" are displayed. These test codes are the default tests for the "CRUDE" sample type.

Press [ESC] when done

```
                    ┌─────────────────────────────┐
                    │                             │
                    │      SAMPLE LOGIN FORM       │
                    │                             │
                    │      SAMPLE NUMBER 5         │
┌───────────────────┴─────────────────────────────┴──────────┐
│                                                             │
│   SUBMISSION NUMBER 2                                       │
│                                                             │
│   SAMPLE NAME                                               │
│   LOCATION                                                  │
│   DUE DATE                                                  │
│   GROUP                                                     │
│   SUBMITTER                                                 │
│   DEPARTMENT                                                │
│   PROJECT                                                   │
│   SOURCE OF SAMPLE                                          │
│   PRIORITY                                                  │
│   COMMENTS                                                  │
│   SAMPLE TYPE                                               │
│                                                             │
└─────────────────────────────────────────────────────────────┘
```

Figure 5-4. PE-Nelson RLAB II sample LOGIN screen. (Nelson Analytical, Inc. 1986. *RLAB II User's Manual.* Cuptertino, Calif. p. 6-2)

```
┌─────────────────────────────────────────────────────────────────────┐
│  MS711                                                               │
│                                              12/01/86      16:11     │
│                        SAMPLE SUBMISSION - SUBMITTER DATA            │
│                        ----------------------------------            │
│   TYPE OF SAMPLE :  EXAMPLE                                          │
│                                                                     │
│   1) SUBMITTER ID       :      NEW                                   │
│   2) STATUS(A/D)        :      .                                     │
│   3) SUBMITTER NAME     :      ....................                  │
│   4) ADDRESS            :      ..............................        │
│                         :      ..............................        │
│                         :      ..............................        │
│   5) PHONE NO.          :      ...............                       │
│   6) DEPT. CODE         :      .....                                 │
│   7) SECTION CODE       :      .....                                 │
│   A)   TYPE AN "X" NEXT TO SELECTED MAIL TYPE. FILL IN ANY ASSOCIATED FIELDS. │
│        SEL    MAIL TYPE                                              │
│                                                                     │
│         .      MAIL                                                  │
│         .      PRINTER - PRINTER CLASS :  .                          │
│         .      PROFS   - PROFS ID      :  ........   USERS NODE:  ........ │
│   B)  GO TO REMOTE SCREEN(Y/N) ?          N                         │
│                                                                     │
│   PF 1=HELP           2=CONTINUE         3=END          10=SELECT    │
└─────────────────────────────────────────────────────────────────────┘
```

Figure 5-5. AXIOM VM LIMS sample LOGIN screen — submitter data. (AXIOM SYSTEMS, Inc. 1988. *VM LIMS Reference Manual User Functions.* East Meadow, N.Y. p. 8-SS)

```
PERKIN-ELMER LIMS 2000                                              ENTER
PAGE 01
01 - SAMPLE NUMBER : R6
02 - PRIORITIZATION : 0              03 - ROUTING : N
04 - DATE PROMISED : 01/25/87
05 - PROJECT CODE : CRUDE           06 - SAMPLE TYPE : 01
07 - LOCATION : LOT 1501
08 - SUBMITTER : RSD                09 - CHARGE NUMBER : 1234

10 - SAMPLE DESCRIPTION : CRUDE SAMPLE
11 - CASE :

PERKIN-ELMER LIMS 2000                                              ENTER
                                   REQUIRED ANALYSIS

ITEM   TEST #      SVC GRP    # REPS      TEST DESCRIPTION
01     RESID       WM         1           RESIDUE AFTER DRYING 1 HR @ 105 DEG C
02     FLASH       RM         1           FLASH POINT (CLOSED CUP)
03     VISC        GN         1           VISCOSITY MEASUREMENT
04     SULFR       GN         1           TOTAL SULFUR IN METALS BY LECO ANALYZER
05     D2887       GC         1           SIMULATED DISTILLATION (ASTM D-2887)
06
```

Figure 5-6. PE-Nelson LIMS 2000 sample LOGIN screen page 1 at top, test descriptions at bottom. (Perkin-Elmer Corp. 1987. *LIMS 2000 Application Programs Manual.* Norwalk, Conn. pp. 1-4,1-5)

Using default test codes saves LIMS sample submitters a lot of time by requiring them to type in one response instead of many. Figure 5-1 indicates which of the comparison LIMS packages offer this feature.

Barcode Labels

The integration of barcode labels into LIMS sample processing is, to put it conservatively, a revelation. The magnitude of time savings achieved by using barcode labels is surpassed only by that of automated test results entry, described in Chapter 7.

There are two primary methods of using barcode labels in association with sample LOGIN. They are related to when, in relation to sample LOGIN, the labels are printed. One method uses preprinted barcode labels; the other method prints a label containing the information entered during sample LOGIN.

Preprinted Barcode Labels.   Figure 5-7 illustrates a sheet of preprinted barcode labels which contains examples of information to be entered during sample LOGIN. Included are user IDs, account (or charge) numbers, test codes, and others. When the sample submitter fills out the sample LOGIN screen, instead of keying in information, he or she can use these barcode. For example, instead of using the keyboard to enter "ASH" or "DSC" into the desired test field of the LOGIN form, the submitter can use an attached barcode wand or laser reader to scan the

Bar Codes for LIMS Commands and Fields
PEL Submitter Version

Figure 5-7. Preprinted barcode labels used to assist a LIMS user In filling out LIMS screens.

entry. Scanning the barcode label is much faster than keying the data manually and eliminates the possibility of character transcription error. A submitter's name (or user ID) will not change. Most sample submitters repeatedly submit the same sample types for the same tests. A label sheet customized for each sample submitter can be provided, containing barcode labels of the responses which are repeatedly used for sample LOGIN. The sheet can be kept near a terminal with an attached barcode reader. Figure 5-8 shows a laser barcode scanner connected to a terminal. The scanner connects between the keyboard and the main terminal unit.

Figure 5-9 also illustrates the use of preprinted barcode labels for a LIMS operation other than sample LOGIN. This illustration, taken from a PE-NELSON ACCESS*LIMS manual (44), is described as "the direct weight measurement bar code command sequence." By entering commands using these barcodes instead of typing them at the keyboard, sample handling time can be greatly reduced.

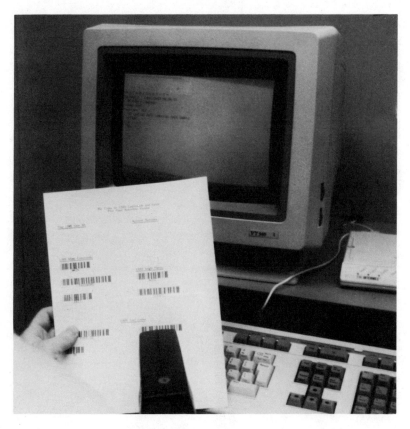

Figure 5-8. Computer terminal with attached barcode reader.

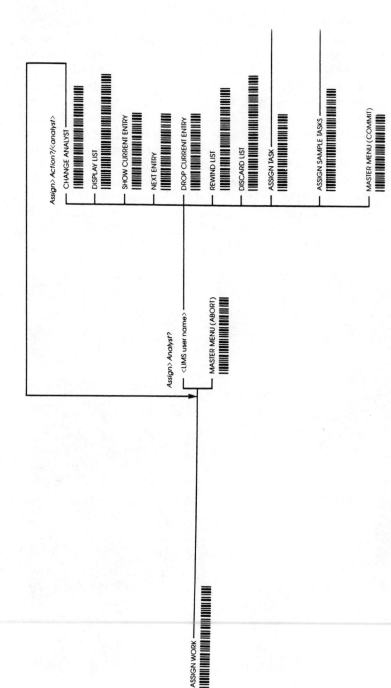

Figure 5-9. Barcode labels used to assist a LIMS user with terminal use.

Sample ID is probably the minimum information needed to accompany a sample as it leaves its origination point on route to the testing lab. Barcode labels containing sets of unique sample IDs can be preprinted on peel-off label stock. When a sample is created, a preprinted label can be placed on the sample container (either a vial or envelope). Then when the sample ID is entered into the LIMS, a barcode reader can be used to scan the sample container instead of using the terminal keyboard to key in the result. Again, barcode entry is faster than using the keyboard and eliminates errors. The preprinted sample ID labels can be in any sequence or form which is used by the sample submitter. They can contain lot numbers, notebook numbers, etc. Figure 5-10 shows another type of preprinted labels.

Barcode Labels Printed by Sample LOGIN.   Some LIMS packages can print barcode labels containing the sample ID, required tests, and anything else that might be required, as a part of the sample LOGIN function. The use of labels printed in this manner can be very flexible because there is no need to use predesignated IDs. After the label is printed, it is attached to the sample container. Subsequent sample handling can then use automated techniques to identify the sample. Figure 5-11 shows which of our comparison LIMS packages offer barcode printing capability.

Access to User-Written Code during Sample LOGIN

Note that although all of the LIMS packages don't specifically offer barcode label printing, it may still be possible to implement this feature through the execution of user-written code. An interface to barcode printing is one reason why it is desirable to have access to your own code during sample LOGIN. Figure 5-11 indicates which LIMS packages offer this access. The use of user-written code to augment the LIMS standard LOGIN function constitutes customization of the system. Customization is discussed in detail in Chapter 12.

Other purposes of user-written code during sample LOGIN are as follows:

1. Interface to the instrument management system to schedule sample processing.
2. Interface to the billing system in order to bill sample submitters for analytical work.
3. Extra security checks on user IDs, sample types, etc.

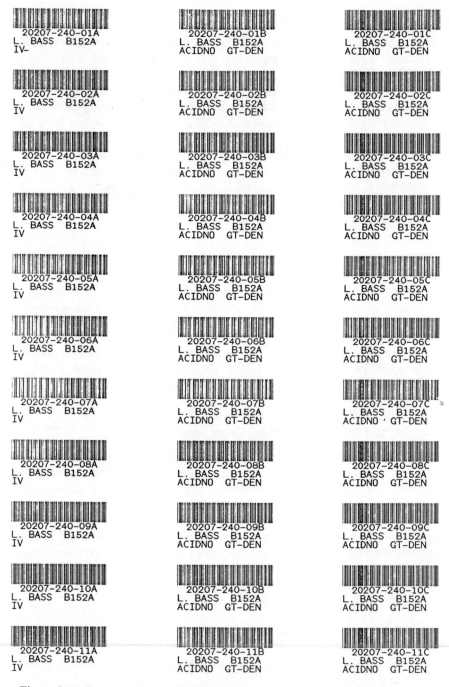

Figure 5-10. Preprinted barcode labels used to attach to sample container. (PE-Nelson Systems, Inc. 1988. *System Specification For ACCESS*LIMS*. Cuptertino, Calif. p. 46)

	A X I O M	B EC CA KL MS A N	L I DM ES C / S M	L A HB PS A M	N ER PLL ESA OB N	2 P0 E0 0	NA EC PLC ESE OS NS	V L A I RM I S A / ND M	S M S A VMN GP A L G E E R
Barcode label printing	X	X	X	X		X	X	X	X
Print extra labels	X	X	X	X		X	X	X	X
Access to user-written code during sample LOGIN		X	X	X		X	X	X	X

Figure 5-11. LIMS comparison — barcode and LOGIN related.

4. Automatic communication with the testing lab indicating that the sample is on its way.
5. Extra help screens.

Collection Lists

"A collection list is a list of samples that are due to be collected and delivered to the laboratory for testing" (46). The following are associated with a collection list:

1. Collector — the person responsible for the collecting the samples comprising the collection list.
2. Collection route — the route, followed by the collector, with stops where samples are to be collected.
3. Dates and times — used to determine which samples are eligible to be collected.

To be included on a collection list, samples must be located on the list's route, must have a date drawn that falls within the dates and times of the list, and must already be logged into the LIMS.

Collection lists are merely information management tools. They are useful to the physical and analytical testing laboratories that collect samples at designated times. They can also be used in areas where samples are produced at regular intervals and delivered to the lab. The use of collection lists is optional. Figure 5-12 shows which of the comparison LIMS packages offer this function.

	A X I O M	B EC CA KL MS A N	L I DM ES C/ S M	L A HB PS A M	N ER PLL ESA OB N	2 P0 E0 0		NA EC PLC ESE OS NS	VL AI RM IS A/ ND M	SM SA VMN GPA LG EE R
Collection list		X	X					X		X

Figure 5-12. LIMS comparison — collection list related.

Summary

We have seen that sample LOGIN is the LIMS function used to input sample information into the LIMS system. This information is needed by the testing laboratory to determine how to process the sample. Required tests and safety information must be known before the sample can be processed. Sample LOGIN is usually performed before analysis, but LOGIN can also follow analysis using a LOGIN-WITH-RESULTS function. This function has the ability to present all sample information to the LIMS, including the test results.

Imaginative integration of barcode labels with LIMS can yield faster processes than were ever achieved with manual, paper methods. If a LIMS user complains that use of the LIMS takes longer than the paper forms that the LIMS replaced, barcode labels may be the answer to this problem.

Chapter 6

Sample RECEIVE, Worksheets, Worklists

Sample RECEIVE

In Chapter 4, we noted that the LIMS sample RECEIVE function follows sample LOGIN in the typical sequence of steps involving the use of a LIMS. We defined sample RECEIVE as: acknowledgment by testing personnel that a sample has been received in the testing laboratory.

Figure 6-1 indicates which LIMS packages offer the RECEIVE function. This function is very important for the LIMS environment where sample creators, as opposed to the testing lab personnel, are expected to log in their own samples. Without this function, the location of the sample can sometimes be unclear. The sample retains a "logged" or "on worksheet" status until a test result is entered. The RECEIVE function changes the sample status from "logged" to "in lab." Thus, by executing the RECEIVE for a particular sample, the testing lab acknowledges receipt of that sample and there is no confusion as to its location. This status change implies a certain responsibility. Although the sample creator, who in many cases is the sample submitter, retains ownership of the sample for its entire lifetime, the responsibility for the sample belongs to the testing lab while it is located there.

The DEC LIMS/SM package provides two methods for receiving samples at the lab: by sample or by collection list. These two methods are illustrated in Figure 6-2. When a sample is received by sample ID, the sample ID is the only entry on the screen. When it is received by collection list, the LIMS/SM package offers the capability to receive several samples at once by filling out one form rather than many.

At the moment the sample RECEIVE function is performed for a given sample, the time is recorded in the LIMS database. At this time, something important happens — a logical timeclock is begun. This timeclock measures the turnaround time for the sample. The turnaround time measurement, which is one of the LIMS supervisory functions discussed in

	A X I O M	B EC CA KL MS A N	L I DM E S C / S M	L A H B P S A M	N ER PLL ESA OB N	2 P0 E0 0	NA EC PLC ESE OS NS	V L A I RM I S A / ND M	M A VN GA G E R
Sample RECEIVE by sample (also called SAMPLING)	X	X	X				X		X
Sample RECEIVE by collection list		X	X						X

Figure 6-1. LIMS comparison — sample RECEIVE related.

Chapter 10, is the time it takes the lab to process the sample. The algorithm used for turnaround time is as follows:

Turnaround time = (time at which the test results are reported to the sample submitter) − (time at which the sample RECEIVE function is performed)

Also, at the moment the sample RECEIVE function is performed, the backlog count is incremented for the tests and/or instruments requested. Counts of backlog used together with turnaround times can be used to manage sample processing in the laboratory. Resource allocation decisions are based on data such as backlogs and turnaround times.

For the majority of the LIMS products without the sample RECEIVE function, the turnaround timeclock begins and the backlog is incremented when the sample is logged. For the LIMS environment requiring sample creators to log their samples using the sample LOGIN function, where there is no RECEIVE function, there is a potential for timing problems. When a sample which has been logged in is delayed in reaching the testing lab for whatever reason, the actual turnaround time for which the lab is responsible will appear needlessly high. Therefore, the concept of the sample RECEIVE function is extremely important when samples are logged by someone other than testing lab personnel.

Worksheets and Worklists

Most LIMS packages offer worklist and/or worksheet functions to assist lab personnel in sample handling. Figure 6-3 indicates which of these functions are offered by the various LIMS packages. Generally, these functions provide lists of samples submitted for testing via sample

```
┌─┬─┬─┬─┬─┬─┐   VAX LIMS/SM
│d│i│g│i│t│a│l│ SAMPLE RECEIVING - BY INDIVIDUAL SAMPLE
└─┴─┴─┴─┴─┴─┘
```

Sample ID: ▮▮▮▮▮▮▮▮▮▮

Date and Time Drawn: 05-MAR-87 10:55:14

Press <PF2> once for HELP on the current field, twice for HELP on the screen

```
┌─┬─┬─┬─┬─┬─┐   VAX LIMS/SM
│d│i│g│i│t│a│l│ SAMPLE RECEIVING - BY COLLECTION LIST
└─┴─┴─┴─┴─┴─┘
```

Route ID: ▮▮▮▮▮▮▮   Collection List ID: ▮▮▮▮▮▮▮

        Sample ID   Date Drawn   Time Drawn   Sample Present
                       05-MAR-87   10:55:19
                       05-MAR-87   10:55:19
                       05-MAR-87   10:55:19
                       05-MAR-87   10:55:19
                       05-MAR-87   10:55:19
                       05-MAR-87   10:55:19
                       05-MAR-87   10:55:19
                       05-MAR-87   10:55:19
                       05-MAR-87   10:55:19
                       05-MAR-87   10:55:19

Press <PF2> once for HELP on the current field, twice for HELP on the screen

Figure 6-2. DEC LIMS/SM sample RECEIVE screen by sample at top, by collection list at bottom.

LOGIN or lists of tests which need to be performed for such samples. Figure 6-4 defines each function, where available, for the various LIMS packages.

As we might expect, the worklist and worksheet functions are similar for most LIMS and identical for some. The major differences lie in organizational characteristics, such as how the sample lists are arranged. For example, the ACCESS*LIMS worklist lists samples which have been assigned to a particular analyst, whereas the LABSAM worklist lists samples which have been assigned to a particular instrument. The LIMS/SM worksheet and the PE LIMS 2000 worklist list samples which have

	A X I O M	B E C C A K L M S A N	L I DM E S C / S M	L A H B P S A M	N ER PLL ESA OB N	2 P0 E0 0	NA EC PLC ESE OS NS	V L A I RM I S A / ND M	M A VN GA G E R
Worklist by analyst	X	X		X	X	X	X	X	X
Worklist by instrument	X	X		X		X	X	X	X
Worklist by test	X	X	X	X	X	X	X	X	X
Worksheet	X	X	X	X				X	X

Figure 6-3. LIMS comparison — worklist/worksheet related.

been submitted for a particular test; the AXIOM worklist provides the same function. The Beckman CALS Lab Manager worklist function lists samples ordered by any parameter associated with the samples or tests.

Figure 6-5 shows the PE LIMS 2000 "wide report" worklist. The worklist can be printed and used by the analyst as a sheet on which to

ACCESS*LIMS
    worklist - list of samples for a particular analyst

AXIOM
    worklist - list of samples for a particular test, instrument, or analyst
    worksheet - used to view sample results

BECKMAN
    worklist - list of samples for a particular sample type, test type, or any
        other parameter associated with the sample

LABSAM
    worklist - list of samples for a particular instrument
    worksheet - list of tests for a particular sample

LIMS/DM
    worklist - list of assigned tests, by workstation, analyst, instrument, or
        combination

LIMS/SM
    worksheet - list of samples for a particular test, by location if desired

PE LIMS 2000
    worklist - list of samples for a particular instrument or analyst

Figure 6-4. Worklist/worksheet definitions.

```
PERKIN-ELMER LIMS 2000                                                        05/04/87 10:55:47
WORKLIST DESCRIPTION DISPLAYED HERE                                                   PAGE 1.01

                                          WORKLIST : AS100
                                          TEST     : AS100

WL#  ID          REP  COPPER  MET  AG  PU  PUAH  TEST FOR  LONGER CAPTION  FE TEST
1    STD1
2    STD2
3    BLANK
4    BLANK
5    SAMP0001 01
6    STD1
7    BLANK
8    SAMP0001 02
9    STD1
10   BLANK
11   SAMP0001 03
12   STD1
13   BLANK
14   SAMP0001 04
15   STD1
16   BLANK
17   SAMP0001 05
18   STD1
19   BLANK
20   SAMP0002 01
21   STD1
22   BLANK
23   SAMP0002 02
24   STD1
25   BLANK
26   SAMP0002 03
```

```
PERKIN-ELMER LIMS 2000                                                        05/04/87 10:55:47
WORKLIST DESCRIPTION DISPLAYED HERE                                                   PAGE 2.01

                                          WORKLIST : AS100
                                          TEST     : AS100

WL#  ID          REP  COPPER  MET  AG  PU  PUAH  TEST FOR  LONGER CAPTION  FE TEST
27   STD1
28   BLANK
29   SAMP0002 04
30   STD1
31   BLANK
32   SAMP0002 05
33   STD1
```

Figure 6-5. PE-Nelson LIMS 2000 wide Report worklist. (Perkin-Elmer Corp. 1987. *LIMS 2000 Application Programs Manual*. Norwalk, Conn. pp. 12-14)

write test results for nonautomated tests. As noted in Chapter 7, some LIMS packages facilitate results entry by providing a "results entry by worklist" function. As with the PE LIMS 2000 system, the results input screen is formatted the same way as the worklist, allowing rapid entry of the data.

Although the LIMS worklist and worksheet functions offered by the various packages are very similar, the differences should be examined closely when choosing a LIMS. If the laboratory prefers to assign samples as they arrive for testing to different analysts based on some criterion such as the analyst's specialty, sample loads, shift requirements, priority, and so on, then a LIMS which creates worklists by analyst would be a valuable tool. For those who may be developing a LIMS, a close evaluation of lab procedures is required to determine which worklist/worksheet type would be most useful.

Summary

Sample RECEIVE capability, as a LIMS function, is important for a laboratory whose customers are expected to submit their own samples using sample LOGIN. Responsibility for the samples is transferred from the sample creator to the testing laboratory by the RECEIVE function. This function also provides a more accurate measurement of turnaround time.

Worksheet and worklist functions provide lists of samples and tests which need to be processed. These functions offered by the various LIMS packages are similar. Differences exist in how the lists of samples and tests are arranged, such as by sample, test, instrument, or analyst. These differences may not appear significant, but they should be examined carefully by those who are writing or selecting a LIMS.

Chapter 7

Test Results Entry

As soon as a physical or analytical test is completed, the test result(s) must be entered into the LIMS. There are two methods of results entry:

1. manual results entry
2. automated results entry

Generally, automated methods of data entry are more accurate, faster, more efficient, and thus desirable whenever possible. The use of manual results entry methods is, however, more prevalent. All commercial LIMS systems have manual results entry capability. Inclusion of automated data entry is made easy with some LIMS, moderately difficult with others, and very difficult with still others.

Manual Results Entry

The manual method of entering anything into a computer is by typing on a terminal keyboard. *Manual results entry* refers to entering test results using the terminal keyboard. This method is initiated by the analyst, or whoever is responsible for entering test results, by instructing the LIMS to perform the manual results entry function. The function displays a form on the screen which is then filled in by the analyst. We should consider the manual method of results entry to be the standard method because it is presented in generally the same form by all LIMS packages. Figure 7-1 lists different methods of manual results entry offered by the various LIMS packages; note that most LIMS offer more than one method. The methods are entry by sample, by test code, by worksheet, and by worklist. Although they are merely variations of the same function, the differences are quite important. Such differences may go unnoticed during evaluations of the various LIMS packages.

As we discuss manual results entry, it is important to remember that many LIMS provide the capability to calculate a final result from a set

	A X I O M	B EC CA KL MS A N	L I DM ES C / S M	L A HB PS A M	N ER PLL ESA OB N	2 P0 E0 0	NA EC PLC ESE OS NS	VL AI RM IS A / ND M	M A VN GA G E R
Results entry by Sample	X	X	X	X		X	X	X	X
Results entry by Test Code	X	X	X		X	X	X		X
Results entry by Worksheet		X	X	X					X
Results entry by Worklist				X		X	X	X	X
Method for final result calculations	X	X	X	X		X		X	X

Figure 7-1. LIMS comparison — test results entry related.

of component data. Calculation algorithms and templates or small segments of user-written code can be predesigned to provide calculations as part of manual result entry. This form of customization is much less flexible than other forms. Thus, although described as manual results entry, calculation of some final results is possible, eliminating manual calculations altogether.

Manual Results Entry by Sample (MRS)

The key entry for the MRS function is the sample ID. After entering the sample ID, the user begins entering test results. Some LIMS prompt the user for each entry, while others provide a form on the terminal screen to fill out. For most LIMS, the MRS function will allow the user to enter test results for all the tests that have been requested for a particular sample. The best use of MRS versus the other methods is when test results need to be entered for only one or two samples or when several tests have been performed on one sample.

Figure 7-2 illustrates the DEC LIMS/SM MRS function. The first entry required from the user is the sample ID. The system then displays all the tests requested for this particular sample. After entering the sample ID, the user begins entering the test results.

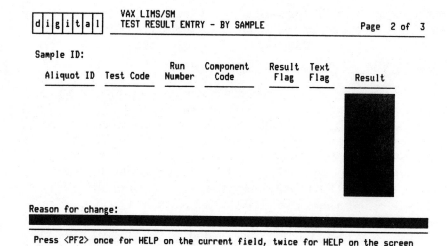

Figure 7-2. DEC LIMS/SM test results entry by sample screen. (Digital Equipment Corporation. 1987. *VAX LIMS/SM Planning Workbook*. Maynard, Mass. p. A-138)

Figure 7-3 illustrates the HP LABSAM MRS function. Again, the first entry required by the user is the sample ID. LABSAM then prompts at the bottom of the screen for a *Test IDC,* which is a specification for a particular test. "When a test IDC is entered, the prompt shown is replaced by the test description, the units of the value, and the input format prompt, all taken from the [previously entered] data specification of the result. The user then enters the value. It is checked against the detection

```
===============================================================================
06/05/84                        RESULT ENTRY BY SAMPLE                 18:32:40
===============================================================================


   SAMPLE    : 84/312
   CUSTOMER  : RANGE 13                     SAMPTYPE   : SLUDGE

   IDC       - P#- M#  Description                  Result      Units
   -------------------------------------------------------------------------
   SB'1                Antimony gravim. (Sb2O4)        3.5      Wt %
   PH                  pH value                       13.9
   Value is above the upper alarm limit by      39.0%
   PB'1      - 1       Lead gravim. (PbSO4)            9.5      Wt %



   Test IDC                    :                        <        IDC,PR#,M#
```

Figure 7-3. HP LABSAM test results entry by sample screen. (Hewlett-Packard Co. 1985. *LABSAM System Reference Manual*. Palo Alto, Calif. p. 4-5)

(if a single result) and alarm limits and the value, together with any messages generated, moves to the top of the screen'' (22).

Manual Results Entry by Test Code (MRT)

When test results are to be entered for a group of samples for the same test, the MRT function is used. The key entry for the MRT function is the Test Code. Use of MRT allows rapid entry of test results for multiple samples. Test results entry with MRT are much faster than with MRS for multiple samples because only one MRT screen is required.

Figure 7-4 illustrates the Perkin Elmer Nelson Systems AC-CESS*LIMS MRT function. The first entry required by the user is the Method, or test name. ''ACCESS*LIMS recognizes four types of result records: NUMBER, TEXT, TIME, and ESSAY. You enter all types of results except ESSAY in the value field of the ENTER METHOD RE-SULTS or ENTER SAMPLE RESULTS form. You enter ESSAY results through the text editor. You can always write text about a result through the text editor'' (45). As the results are entered they are checked against previously determined *measure limits* and *detection limits*. A SUSPECT status is given to results which are found to be outside limits.

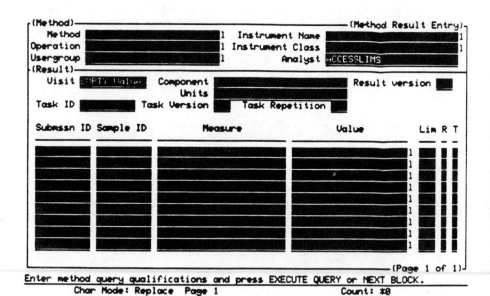

Figure 7-4. PE-Nelson ACCESS*LIMS test results entry by test screen. (PE-Nelson Systems, Inc. 1988. *System Specification For ACCESS*LIMS*. Cuptertino, Calif. p. 47)

The Axiom VM LIMS allows the user to select either MRS or MRT by entering a response on the screen shown in Figure 7-5. If a Test Code is entered, the user will be prompted by a series of *computer-aided testing dialogs*. The dialogs, which are optional, are "predefined prompts and computations that follow the way the actual testing is done in the laboratory. If no dialogues are present for a test method, computer-aided testing will prompt for the final results directly" (27).

Manual Results Entry by Worksheet (MRW)

To enter test results for samples which were previously placed on a worksheet, the MRW function is used. The key entry for this function is the worksheet ID. Use of MRW allows rapid entry of test results for multiple samples processed for the same test or different tests.

Figure 7-6 shows the main menu for the Varian LIMS/DM package. As illustrated, the "Manual Results Entry" has been chosen. The user has been prompted for the name of a worklist containing samples for which results need to be entered, and has entered the worklist name BALANCE ASH. Figure 7-7 shows the worklist, BALANCE ASH, ready for results to be entered for samples 86042800081 and 86042800082. After results have been entered for the components, tare weight, total

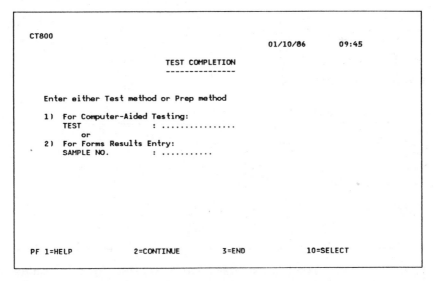

Figure 7-5. AXIOM VM LIMS test completion screen. (AXIOM SYSTEMS, INC. 1988. *VM LIMS Reference Manual Users Functions. East Meadow, N.Y.* p. 3-CT)

```
┌─────────────┐   LIMS/DM
│ v a r i a n │   MAIN MENU
└─────────────┘
```

	Command	Description
^	CONFIGURE	Define LIMS Configuration
I	DAS	Data Analysis System
	DIRECTORY	Record Directories
	EXCEPTION	Exception Handling
	EXIT	Exit LIMS
	INSTRUMENT	Instrument Data Acquisition
	LOGIN	Sample Login
	REPORT	Sample Reports
	RESULTS	Manual Results Entry
	REVIEW	Review Test Results
I	SELECT	Select Tests
v	STATUS	Status Reports

-> Selection: RESULTS

Worklist Name: BALANCE ASH

Figure 7-6. Varian LIMS/DM main menu screen. (Varian Associates. 1986. *Varian Laboratory Data Management User's Manual*. Varian LIMS/DM Version 1.7.1. Walnut Creek, Calif. p. 7-6)

```
┌─────────────┐   LIMS/DM                                    Function
│ v a r i a n │   RESULTS ENTRY
└─────────────┘                          ───── 08-FEB-89 / 10:50 AM
```

Worklist Name: BALANCE ASH   Analyst ID: DEMO

Expected Limits: 90 To 120 grams

No.	Sample ID	Ali	R	Crucible #	Method ID - Section	Component	Result	Comments
1	89020800001	1	1		ASH - SAMPLE	TARE WT.	93.26	
2	89020800001	1	1		ASH - SAMPLE	TOTAL WT.	103.12	
3	89020800001	1	1		ASH - SAMPLE	SAMPLE WT.	9.86	
4	89020800001	1	1		ASH - SAMPLE	FINAL WT.		
5	89020800001	1	1		ASH - SAMPLE	ASH WT.		
6	89020800001	1	1		ASH - SAMPLE	ASH WT%		
7	89020800002	1	1		ASH - SAMPLE	TARE WT.		
8	89020800002	1	1		ASH - SAMPLE	TOTAL WT.		
9	89020800002	1	1		ASH - SAMPLE	SAMPLE WT.		

Figure 7-7. Varian LIMS/DM test results entry by worklist screen. (Varian Associates. 1986. *Varian Laboratory Data Management User's Manual*. Varian LIMS/DM Version 1.7.1. Walnut Creek, Calif. p. 7-7)

weight, sample weight, final weight, and ash weight, the final result which is ash weight percent is calculated automatically.

Automated Results Entry

Over the years, analytical instruments have become more accurate and precise. They have become faster, thus providing the ability to process more and more samples in a given amount of time. Advances in electronics are, of course, primarily responsible. In the early 1970s, computer technology found its way into the laboratory in the form of signal processors, such as integrators, which replaced strip chart recorders on chromatographs and other instrumentation. Eight-bit computers later replaced the integrators and added the ability to process raw data and provide peak areas, compound names, mass numbers, retention times, etc. By the early 1980s, instruments with built-in computers were common. This on-board computing allowed raw data to be processed within the instrument and at the same time facilitated communications to a printer or a multipurpose computer system.

Results which are entered into a LIMS without having to be typed at a terminal keyboard are said to be *automated*. Automated results entry is one purpose for automated laboratory instrumentation (described in Chapter 3) which is composed of data acquisition and instrument management. An instrument-to-computer connection provides the pathway for automatic data transfer into the LIMS. Manual result entry has always been plagued with the entry of wrong numbers and character transcription errors, the latter being the more prevalent error type. As stated above, direct transfer of test results from the instrument to the LIMS is more accurate than manual results entry and completely eliminates both types of errors.

The efficiency gained by automated results entry is tremendous. Many routinely used instruments, such as gas and liquid chromatographs, titrimeters, viscometers, scintillation counters, ultraviolet and atomic absorption spectrometers, and calorimeters, come with computer connections. Many of the more expensive instruments such as X-ray diffractometers, Fourier transfer infrared, nuclear magnetic resonance units, X-ray and mass spectrometers, come with computers on which they rely for data collection and processing. Those instruments with either a computer connection or with attached computer are candidates for interfacing and direct results entry into a LIMS.

Entering results into the LIMS database is usually quicker with automated methods than with manual methods. Of course, if an analyst completes a test and immediately enters the result via a terminal, this may prove quicker than using a computer connection. But over the long run, for large numbers of samples, it is not possible for manual methods to be consistently faster than automated data links. It may be possible to hire enough clerical help to supplement lab analysts for the purpose of enhancing manual data entry. Enough people inputting data manually could approach the speed of an automated instrument, but it would not be cost effective. Figure 7-8 lists features and options associated with automated results entry and instrumentation.

Data Acquisition Systems

The data acquisition system interfaces instruments for the purpose of automated results entry. It consists of a data system, connected to one or more instruments, which is designed to communicate with the LIMS. The data system, of course, is a computer system and may or may not be the system on which the LIMS is running. Varian defines an instrument as follows: "To LIMS/DM, an instrument can be any piece of equipment that sends data to an input/output port of the VAX computer.

	A X I O M	B EC CA KL MS A N	L I DM ES C/ S M	L A HB PS A M	N ER PLL ESA OB N	2 P0 E0 0	NA EC PLC ESE OS NS	VL AI RM IS A/ ND M	M A VN GA G E R
Automated Results Entry	X	X		X	X	X	X	X	X
Interface instruments from other vendors	X	X	X	X		X		X	X
Optional data acquisition/data management options		X		X		X	X	X	X
Instrument Management System option		X						X	
Access user-written code during results entry	X	X	X	X		X		X	X

Figure 7-8. LIMS comparison — results entry related.

This will generally be either an analytical instrument with in-board data handling and communications capabilities, such as the Techtron SpectrAA 20/30 atomic absorption spectrophotometer, or a data station, such as the Varian DS 604, that is in turn connected to an instrument which generates an analog output signal (such as a chromatograph detector signal)'' (47). Each instrument connected to the VAX communicates by using a unique Instrument Management (IM) module. Each IM module is a computer program which is custom written, by either Varian or the user, to communicate via the specific requirements and protocol of the particular instrument. Because there are no communications standards for analytical instrumentation, most IM modules must be different. However, although Varian offers many IM modules as options, they also offer a Generic Interface Module (GIM). The GIM is the first of a continuing effort to take advantage of the few similarities that do exist in instrument-to-computer communications. As new models of instruments are designed, it is likely that they will be easier to interface. The GIM will evolve to become a more useful and a more important tool for laboratory automation.

HP LABSAM interfaces similarly to instruments. "Automatic dialogues differ from instrument to instrument and users must write interpreters to handle the different data strings and formats" (48). The Beckman EDLAB program "provides the necessary link to allow data from LIL (Laboratory Interface Language), other files, or databases to flow into the CALS Lab Manager database" (41). LIL is used to program the Beckman MK5 Digimetry instrument coupler, which provides a distributed interface to lab instruments and barcode devices.

The PE-Nelson ACCESS*LIMS System Specifications manual (29) describes a three step procedure for instrument interfacing:

1. The instrument or data analysis system produces a file containing the test results.
2. Custom or PE-Nelson programs interpret the results file and create an ARE (Automatic Result Entry) file. The ARE file is placed in a shared directory on the ACCESS*LIMS computer.
3. ACCESS*LIMS reads the ARE file and writes the information into the appropriate database records.

The LIMS package sold by instrument vendors will easily interface to their own instruments. Sophisticated systems which offer data management functions are available. HP LABSAM interfaces readily to its Laboratory Automation System (LAS). PE LIMS 2000 interfaces readily to its Chromatography Laboratory Automation System (CLAS). Beckman CALS interfaces readily to its Instrument Data Acquisition System (IDAS). We would expect to interface an instrument vendor's LIMS to instruments from the same vendor with no user-written code. This is generally the case.

Data acquisition systems can be simple or complex. Simple systems communicate only from instrument to computer. When the instrument is ready to communicate, it does. If the computer is not ready for the data, they are lost. More complex systems maintain two-way communications between instrument and computer to synchronize data transfers. Some data acquisition systems, like those mentioned above, also provide extensive additional features such as data management functions. VG's state-of-the-art Multichrom chromatography data acquisition network servers have extended the limits of data acquisition to an unrestricted networked environment (49). VG's Ethernet networking scheme may seem complex compared to many instrument interfaces, but it will soon be commonplace and viewed as simple. PE-Nelson's AC-CESS*CHROM system "is a multi-tasking, multi-user chromatography system designed for analytical laboratories that need a centralized approach to chromatography data processing" (50). ACCESS*CHROM, an example of excellent software, is compatible with ACCESS*LIMS for data acquisition. ACCESS*CHROM is also designed to be used on a distributed local area Ethernet network by connecting to interfaces which attach to Ethernet terminal servers.

Interfacing instruments to either the LIMS host computer or a smaller lab computer is not difficult or expensive. In Figure 7-8, all the LIMS interface to instruments. Simple programming/interfacing techniques are used to read data from instruments. If this capability doesn't exist in house, it can be readily obtained either from the LIMS vendor or from firms offering contract programming specifically for laboratory automation (32). As described in Chapter 15, in purchasing a LIMS, one must be aware that additional work is required to customize it to the lab's environment. And this additional work includes instrument interfacing. There are no technological impediments to automating laboratories. Laboratory computer support groups are becoming more skilled at interfacing instruments, and instrument vendors are making it easier with each new model. Thus, relative to the benefit gained, instrument interfacing is not expensive.

Instrument Management System

By using a LIMS in the laboratory, one can manage many more types of information than ever before. Accompanying automated results entry is instrument management. Any time we consider automated results entry in the laboratory we must also consider instrument management. What is instrument management? Organizationally, as described in Chapter 3, instrument management is part of automated laboratory instrumentation, which is part of laboratory automation. Functionally, instrument management is concerned with any activity or data related to the use of an instrument. More accurately, instrument management done in conjunction with a LIMS should be called *automated instrument management*. Either way, instrument management has one primary objective: the use of an instrument which can be proven to produce accurate and precise results.

Of course, the reason for obtaining accurate and precise results is obvious, but as previously indicated, we must be able to prove it. For example, "not only must a regulated laboratory produce quality data, but that data itself can be invalidated if an instrument has not been properly calibrated or maintained or if accurate records of these operations are not retained and available." Continuing, Beckman Instruments states that "the CALS Lab Manager System provides an effective, fully automated solution to these requirements" (28). Thus, this is an example of the use of an instrument management system as part of a LIMS, as documented in Figure 7-8.

Communications Standards

As stated above, there are no communications standards for laboratory instrumentation. Standards to facilitate instrument interfacing might actually consist of some very simple rules and implementation guidelines. First, an ASCII communications standard might be keyword driven. An analytical instrument could be sent the command "BEGIN" from an attached computer. Then, the first keyword from the instrument could be "START", followed by any number of keywords and data items, in any order. The format of the data items might be the same for each general category of instruments. Once all the data has been sent by the instrument, it could send an "ENDDATA" message to the computer.

Of course this description may be lacking in needed functionality such as data verification and error checking, but it is important to remember that communications between an instrument and a computer do not have to be complicated. In fact, the simpler the better. Most sophisticated instrumentation come with built-in or added-on computers and are capable of providing most of the required data reduction. Data from less complicated instrumentation are usually less complicated and are generally fairly easy to communicate to an attached computer. A few simple communication standards could greatly enhance laboratory automation.

Standards organizations such as ASTM are committed to addressing laboratory communications standards. They will define universal standards which will enable simple instrument interfacing. In the future, to interface a laboratory instrument to a LIMS, an analyst will have to connect the instrument to the computer and indicate the following to the LIMS: (1) the computer port number, such as "TXA1", and (2) the type of instrument, such as "GC."

Access to User-Written Code during Results Entry

As shown in Figure 7-8, some LIMS packages provide access to user-written code during results entry. This feature is extremely useful in calculating and verifying final results, comparing results against standards, accessing calibration data, and also in interfacing instruments, other computers, and other software systems. For example, assume that a lab is using a titrimeter controlled by a PC. The following sample processing sequence employs user-written code during results entry:

1. A sample is analyzed on the titrimeter.
2. The raw data are collected by the PC.
3. Results are calculated from the raw data by the PC titration program and stored in a PC disk file.
4. A terminal emulator/file transfer program, such as KERMIT, is used to transfer the result file to the LIMS host.
5. The analyst runs the LIMS *results entry function* and begins to enter data for the sample.
6. The analyst is prompted for the name of the file containing the titration results which have been transferred from the PC.
7. The analyst enters the file name, which is passed to a user-written subroutine.
8. The subroutine parses the titration results from the file and returns them to LIMS.

This is a very simple method to interface data acquisition to the LIMS. Accessing user-written code constitutes customization of the LIMS and is discussed further in Chapter 12.

Summary

Test results entry is a major function of the LIMS. It is accomplished in a variety of ways by the various LIMS packages. Manual results entry can be organized into several differently sorted groupings, such as by worksheet or test code. Automated results entry makes use of computer-instruments links and data acquisition systems. Data acquisition systems can be very simple and provide only data transfer, or they can be multifeatured systems which include data management. Instrument management systems are needed to help us ensure that our instruments are performing to the best of their ability.

Chapter 8

Result Verification and Reporting Results

Result Verification

In most instances, when using a LIMS, we expect to review test results by looking at them on a LIMS screen and indicating either approval or disapproval. This is the manual method of review. Some LIMS packages allow automatic review of test results. We will first examine the manual method of result review and then look at automatic methods.

Manual Result Verification

After all test results for a sample have been completed and entered into the LIMS, and after all calculations and data reductions have been completed, the next step is *result verification,* sometimes referred to as *result validation.* Any sample information must be verified, or reviewed, before it leaves the testing lab. In most cases, result verification is not done to question the ability of lab members but only to guard against simple mistakes. The most common mistakes are the following:

Character transcription errors; for example, the value 157 might be entered for 175
Reporting sample A's results with sample B, and vice versa
Failure to detect an out-of-limits condition

The decision as to who is authorized to verify results is usually left up to the lab manager. A senior analyst or senior lab technician may be authorized to review results, or the lab manager may be the only person authorized to do so. In some laboratories, the analyst who actually completed the work performs the review. Two levels of review are sometimes required — the first level perhaps by the analyst who completed the test, followed by approval from the manager or a senior lab member.

Very elaborate review systems have evolved in some laboratories as a result of dedication to quality output and service. The problem is that verification of results takes time. As the labs process more and more samples with fewer human resources, the percentage of time required for verification, based on the laboratory as a whole, increases dramatically. For example, assume that an analyst processing GC samples 10 years ago had access to five chromatographs and that each sample required a run time of 20 minutes. Allowing for sample preparation time, result verification time, and sending out result reports, the analyst might process about 75 samples per day. Assume that today the analyst still has five chromatographs, each with autosamplers and capable of processing the samples with 10-minute run times. The analyst could easily process 150 samples per day. The total analysis time requirement has remained the same, but the result verification time requirement has doubled.

As more and more computing technology is integrated into the laboratory, how might electronic information management techniques be used to help reduce the time requirement for results verification? A LIMS presents lists of samples and test results which can be quickly viewed by the result reviewer. By using this review function, the reviewer can agree with the test results, disagree with them, call for a retest of the sample, or even cancel the sample. A LIMS is designed to streamline the review process. The various LIMS packages offer several methods by which samples can be sorted to facilitate review. These include sorting by project, by study, by sample ID, by date, by submitter, by collection list, by worksheet, and others. Figure 8-1 indicates the review options offered by our comparison set of LIMS packages.

Figure 8-2 illustrates the Varian LIMS/DM "Review Test Results — Selection" screen form. By using this form, the LIMS user can fill in any combination of fields in order to retrieve selected samples for review. For example, "if you want to review only those test results which have been completed since March 20, 1986 by an analyst named Cooper using a LIMS/DM method called AROMATICS, you would enter N into the All:Y/N field, 03-20-86 into the Starting Date Analyzed field, COOPER into the analyst ID field, and AROMATICS into the Method ID field. Only those tests with matching entries in all three fields would be retrieved" (47).

Figure 8-3 shows the DEC LIMS/SM "Test Result Review — By Test Code" screen. If the LIMS user wanted to review all completed results for an elemental analysis test with a LIMS/SM test code name "CHN," the user would enter "CHN" in the Test Code field. All samples and aliquots with a "CO," or completed, test status would then be displayed, as shown in Figure 8-4. The user would then enter an Action Code in

	AXIOM	BECKLMSAN	LIDMESC/SM	LAHBPSAM	NERPLLESAOBN	2P0E00	NAECPLCESEOSNS	VLAIRMISA/NDM	SMSAVMNGPALGEER
Review results by project		X		X	X				
Review by batch	X	X		X				X	
Review by instrument		X						X	
Review by sample source		X		X				X	
Review by sample type	X	X		X	X		X	X	
Review results by study		X			X		X		X
Review results by submission	X	X			X		X		
Review results by sample ID	X	X	X	X	X	X	X	X	X
Review results by date		X		X	X			X	
Review results by submitter		X		X				X	X
Review results by worksheet		X	X	X				X	X
Review by test code	X	X	X		X			X	X
Multiple levels of results review	X	X	X						X
Automatic validation	X	X		X	X	X	X	X	X
Reason for change required after results review	X	X		X		X	X	X	X

Figure 8-1. LIMS comparison — results review.

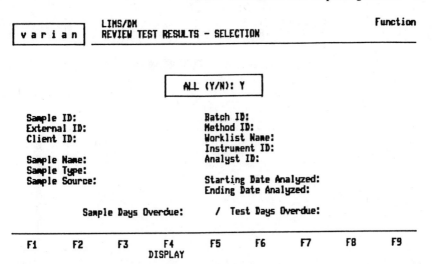

Figure 8-2. Varian LIMS/DM review test results — selection screen. (Varian Associates. 1986. *Varian Laboratory Data Management User's Manual.* Varian LIMS/DM Version 1.7.1. Walnut Creek, Calif. p. 9-3)

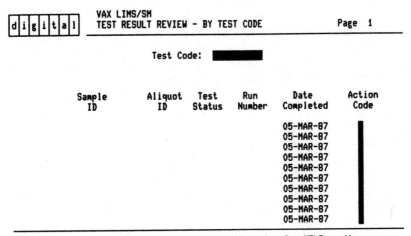

Figure 8-3. DEC LIMS/SM test result review — by test code screen. (Digital Equipment Corp. 1987. *VAX LIMS/SM Planning Workbook.* Maynard, Mass. p. A-152)

```
┌─┬─┬─┬─┬─┬─┬─┐   VAX LIMS/SM V1.1                                    FUNCTION
│d│i│g│i│t│a│l│   TEST RESULT REVIEW - BY TEST CODE              Page  1 of  3
└─┴─┴─┴─┴─┴─┴─┘
```

Test Code: ▓CHN▓▓▓▓▓

Sample ID	Aliquot ID	Test Status	Run Number	Date Completed	Action Code
LIMS-TEST-1	P	CO	1	14-DEC-88	U
LIMS-TEST-2	P	CO	1	14-DEC-88	U
LIMS-TEST-3	P	CO	1	14-DEC-88	U
				- -	
				- -	
				- -	
				- -	
				- -	

Press <PF2> once for HELP on the current field, twice for HELP on the screen

Figure 8-4. Test result review — by test code for CHN test code, page 1.

the action code field. The action codes consist of a single letter as follows: (1) A — agree, (2) D — disagree, (3) R — retest, or (4) U — unreview. If the user enters an "R," the test is resubmitted and the run number is incremented. To look at actual test results, the user places the cursor on the desired line and presses the Next Page function key. Page 2 of the form, shown in Figure 8-5, is then displayed. Scanning results in this manner can be very efficient because the reviewer need only look for out-of-limit flags. If no flags exist, the reviewer can quickly advance to the next sample. Looking for error flags instead of looking at each result is a means of *reviewing by exception*. The user can look at the limits for a particular test component by moving the cursor to the desired line and pressing the Next Page function key. The limits are then displayed on page 3 of the form, shown in Figure 8-6.

Automatic Result Verification

As indicated in Figure 8-1, some LIMS packages offer the ability to review test results automatically. These methods are very similar to manual methods and illustrate how a LIMS can be tailored to speed sample processing. The HP LABSAM automatic method works during result entry by checking "the validation level of the person who enters the result. If this level equals or exceeds that required by the test, the result is flagged finally validated" (48).

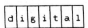

```
              VAX LIMS/SM V1.1                              FUNCTION
              TEST RESULT DISPLAY                    Page  2 of  3


         Sample ID:  LIMS-TEST-1      Aliquot ID:  P

         Test Code:  CHN              Date Received:  14-DEC-88

         Run Number:  1

            Component       Test        Result     Limit
              Code         Result        Units    Test Flag

            CARBON          20            %                     ▌
            HYDROGEN        25            %
            NITROGEN        30            %




    _____
    Press <PF2> once for HELP on the current field, twice for HELP on the screen
```

Figure 8-5. Test result review — by test code for CHN test code, test result display.

```
              VAX LIMS/SM V1.1                              FUNCTION
              TEST RESULT DETAILS DISPLAY           Page  3 of  3


         Sample ID:  LIMS-TEST-1          Aliquot ID:  P

         Test Code:  CHN                  Date Received:  14-DEC-88
         Run Number:  1

         Units:          %               Component Code:  CARBON
         High Valid Limit:      100
         High Limit:            100       Test Result:     20
         Low Limit:               0
         Low Valid Limit:         0       Limit Test Flag:

   Result Text:



    _____
    Press <PF2> once for HELP on the current field, twice for HELP on the screen
```

Figure 8-6. Test result review — by test code for CHN test code, test result details display.

The PE-NELSON RLAB automatic review method is similar to the DEC LIMS/SM manual method described above and illustrated in Figures 8-3 and 8-4. A list of completed samples is displayed and can be verified without actually seeing the results. (The DEC LIMS/SM results can be viewed by advancing to page 2 of the form.)

The purposes of the automatic methods are certainly not to shortcut GLP guidelines. One form of automatic verification in a lab consists of entering test results into the LIMS from an IM system. If the results have already been examined on the IM before transfer to the LIMS and verified as correct, there is no reason to verify them a second time in a LIMS verification step.

Generally, most LIMS can be operated at whatever result verification level is best suited to the laboratory operation. Either multiple verification steps or none at all can be required. The purpose of results verification is to maintain high-quality output. If it can be done externally from the LIMS, or in some other fashion related to results entry, then there is no need for a redundant verification step. But in most instances, result verification should be considered mandatory, and the LIMS can help to enforce this requirement.

Reporting Results

Reporting test results to the sample submitter is a major LIMS function. Test results are eligible for reporting as soon as they are verified. Several methods of reporting results are available. They include standard results reports, ad hoc reporting, and automatic results reporting. Most LIMS packages come with a standard report format which is produced by executing the results report function. Electronic report delivery is also offered by some LIMS packages. Figure 8-7 indicates the sorting options offered by the LIMS comparison set.

Standard Results Reports

Most commercial LIMS packages, and even those written in house, present a standard results report format (or formats) to the LIMS user. After the test results for a sample or group of samples have been entered and verified, a lab member produces the results report by running the results report function. The report is either printed on the lab's printer and put in the plant mail to the sample submitter or printed on a printer in another location (perhaps closer to the sample submitter if external to the lab), or the report is sent via electronic mail to the submitter's computer mail account.

	A X I O M	B EC CA KL MS A N	L I DM E S C / S M	L A H B P S A M	N ER PLL ESA OB N	2 P0 E0 0	NA EC PLC ESE OS NS	VL AI RM I S A / ND M	SM SA VMN GPA LG EE R
Results report by sample ID	X	X	X	X	X	X	X	X	X
Results report by project		X	X	X	X	X	X		X
Results report by submitter		X	X	X	X	X	X		X
Results report by date		X	X	X	X	X	X		X
Results report by worklist		X				X	X		X
Results report by batch	X	X		X	X	X	X		X
Results report by study (sub)	X	X	X		X	X	X		X
Results report by test code		X			X	X	X	X	
Variable report formats		X	X	X	X	X	X		X
Report delivery to printer	X	X	X	X	X	X	X	X	X
Report delivery to file	X	X	X	X	X	X	X	X	X
Report delivery via elec. mail	X	X	X				X	X	X
Results interface available to external packages such as LOTUS, RS/1, SAS	X	X	X		X	X	X	X	X

Figure 8-7. LIMS comparison — results report.

For some LIMS, the standard formats are very limited in what can be specified to go on the report, while for others, there is great flexibility. Figure 8-8 shows the DEC LIMS/SM results report screen. As noted on the last line of the form, a report format can be entered. Figure 8-9 illustrates a report produced by filling out the form, specifying a "printer" report type and the default report format. The "default" report format is the only one delivered with the LIMS/SM product, for which the vendor does include the FORTRAN source code. The vendor intends this program to be a model which the customer can use to design additional formats.

Ad Hoc Reporting

The capability to provide ad hoc database searching in order to produce reports of analytical data is an extremely powerful LIMS feature. Ad hoc searching means that the searcher is not restricted to a relatively few search criteria. No matter how much planning goes into the design of report formats and the search structure, someone will always want to retrieve data in an unusual or unanticipated manner. As illustrated above, the users of some LIMS packages can design an unlimited number of reports using programming languages, but this is not ad hoc searching. The concept of ad hoc searching also implies a relative ease of use.

The use of SQL search techniques, described in Chapter 4, provides a high level of user friendliness. PE-Nelson's ACCESS*LIMS provides

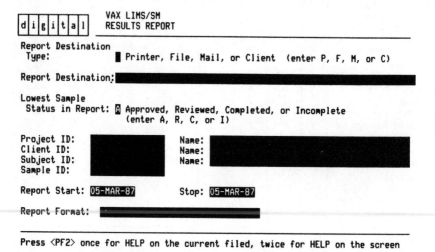

Figure 8-8. DEC LIMS/SM results report screen. (Digital Equipment Corp. 1987. *VAX LIMS/SM Planning Workbook.* Maynard, Mass. p. 9-26)

```
14-DEC-1988 13:02

Sample ID: LIMS-TEST-1    , P  ,    1
Test: CHN          (Elemental Analysis for C, H, & N)
Results Entered By:  LIMS System Manager                    14-Dec-1988
Results Reviewed By: LIMS System Manager                    14-Dec-1988
   Component          Component Description                 Result
  ----------  ------------------------------------------  -----------------
   CARBON      Weight % Carbon                       20        %
   HYDROGEN    Weight % Hydrogen                     25        %
   NITROGEN    Weight % Nitrogen                     30        %

Sample ID: LIMS-TEST-2    , P  ,    1
Test: CHN          (Elemental Analysis for C, H, & N)
Results Entered By:  LIMS System Manager                    14-Dec-1988
Results Reviewed By: LIMS System Manager                    14-Dec-1988
   Component          Component Description                 Result
  ----------  ------------------------------------------  -----------------
   CARBON      Weight % Carbon                       21        %
   HYDROGEN    Weight % Hydrogen                     26        %
   NITROGEN    Weight % Nitrogen                     31        %

Sample ID: LIMS-TEST-3    , P  ,    1
Test: CHN          (Elemental Analysis for C, H, & N)
Results Entered By:  LIMS System Manager                    14-Dec-1988
Results Reviewed By: LIMS System Manager                    14-Dec-1988
   Component          Component Description                 Result
  ----------  ------------------------------------------  -----------------
   CARBON      Weight % Carbon                       22        %
   HYDROGEN    Weight % Hydrogen                     27        %
   NITROGEN    Weight % Nitrogen                     32        %
```

Figure 8-9. Results report for three samples.

SQL capability by making use of a third-party relational database product. ACCESS*LIMS is built around the use of the Oracle database. The Oracle products include several options for queries and graphics. ACCESS*LIMS includes some of the Oracle options upon which its reporting capability is based. The following is an example SQL session which illustrates an ad hoc database search. This search is constructed to help isolate the cause of a problem: an unusual number of control samples for a particular test have been flagged as out of range. SQL is used to query the database to retrieve information in a meaningful manner. A report is generated containing sample IDs, result values, and the instrument IDs for all control types STANDARDTHM where the out of range flag is set.

```
SELECT SAMPLE, RESULT, INSTRUMENT
   FROM CONTROL_RESULTS
   WHERE CONTROL_TYPE = 'STANDARDTHM' AND
      RESULT_OUT_RANGE IS NOT NULL
   ORDER BY INSTRUMENT, DATE_TIME_ENTERED
```

Other examples of external interfaces for test results which are provided by LIMS packages are the PE-Nelson RLAB-to-Lotus 123 interface and the DEC LIMS/SM-to-RS/1 interface.

Automatic Results Reporting

The HP LABSAM system allows up to 200 different report formats to be predefined by the user. Even more useful is LABSAM's automatic results reporting, triggered when a sample status reaches final validation (48). Thus, upon final validation of a sample, the sample's test results are automatically printed without having to run a reporting function separately. Automatic results reporting is a very useful feature because it eliminates a step from the sample processing sequence. It has been demonstrated that other LIMS packages can be customized to produce results reports automatically as part of the result verification step.

Summary

Result verification is a function offered by LIMS packages as a means of reviewing test results before they leave the lab. Verification can often be streamlined to fit the lab's procedures. It can also be automated or eliminated. On the one hand, elimination of result verification may lower the quality of lab output. On the other hand, if quality is built into the testing procedures in the first place, the need for result verification can be eliminated. Automated instrumentation and automated data collection by the LIMS goes a long way toward eliminating data handling errors.

The test results of a sample are usually reported by the lab after completing the test(s) and verifying the results. LIMS packages offer various report formats and methods to sort test results. Automating the results reporting function is possible and should be considered a must by any organization using LIMS. The use of proprietary databases designed specifically for the LIMS product may become the atypical choice of LIMS vendors in the future. Some current LIMS packages are being designed around commercial database products which offer many extra searching and reporting features.

Section Three

Using, Choosing, and Managing

Chapter 9

LIMS Setup

The previous chapters in Section Two have examined the various LIMS functions. Comparisons of commercial LIMS functions have been used to illustrate the use of and differences between the functions. In Chapter 10 we will describe the LIMS supervisory functions. As we've seen thus far, the purpose of a LIMS package is to manage sets of data and information about users, samples, test methods, sample types, instrument types, and other things found in a laboratory environment.

Each commercial LIMS package has a different nomenclature for its operating data. Axiom's VM LIMS keeps its operating data, which it calls *static data,* in a set of *dictionaries* (27). The data consists of the following:

Employee access	Employee information
Department code	Section code
Account number	Project link code
Priority	Handling codes
Printer	Disposal
Profs	Remark code
Note code	Result code
Test code	Group test
Submitter access	

DEC's LIMS/SM maintains a similar set of data upon which it operates (54). These data are described as:

Test	Test group
Sample type	Schedule
Location	Collections route
Collector	User
System mapping	Test mapping
Client	Project
Subject	Device and instrument type

Routine, day-to-day operation of the LIMS requires upkeep of these data and information in order to include new users, tests, etc., in the system. Before a system can be used for the first time, an initial set of these items must be defined. For example, the Varian LIMS/DM system requires configuration of worklists, method sections, method procedures, privileges, user accounts, terminal accounts, and instruments. It is important to remember that LIMS are not simply plugged in and used. The purpose of this chapter is to stress two important aspects of LIMS setup, preinstallation planning, and security. Detailed planning is required before beginning a LIMS installation, as discussed in detail in Chapter 11. The perceived value of analytical information will vary among LIMS installations, but in most cases, too much attention cannot be given to LIMS security considerations.

Preinstallation Planning

Planning for setup of the initial parameters is done before the system is installed. Sizing the LIMS database may actually depend on the results of this planning; thus, accurate planning is required. If an evaluation was conducted prior to software selection, much of the information necessary for the initial setup of the LIMS will be readily available. Chapter 11 describes the determination of system requirements and preselection planning, which refers to planning done before selecting a LIMS. Initial evaluations of laboratories, tests, samples, customers, users, data end use, instrumentation, and reports will provide the information necessary for LIMS setup.

Some LIMS packages provide *planning workbooks* to help LIMS managers with the initial setup. Of course, the vendors will make available whatever services are required during setup, either included in the purchase or as an option. In fact, Beckman advertises that they "begin the installation process before you place your order" by helping you "define your system precisely" (57).

The DEC *VAX LIMS/SM Planning Workbook* (52) provides a set of charts which are to be filled out before installation. These charts help LIMS managers to collect the information necessary to configure the LIMS initially. These charts include the following:

Clients Chart	Data-Reduction Algorithms
Collection Routes Chart	Chart
Collectors Chart	Data Storage Requirements
Computer Equipment Chart	Chart

Devices Chart
Help-Screen Tailoring
    Chart
ID Algorithms Chart
Instrument Types Chart
Locations Chart
Menu Changes Chart
Parameters Chart
Projects Chart
Quick Reference Sheet
    for Clients
Quick Reference Sheet
    for Group Test Codes
Quick Reference Sheet
    for Projects
Quick Reference Sheet
    for Subjects

Quick Reference Sheet
    for Test Codes
Sample Types Chart
Schedules Chart
Screen Tailoring Chart
Specific Tests, Test Limits
    Chart
Subjects Chart
Summary Sheet of Customized
    Screens
Summary of Tailored Screens
Test Chart
Test Group Chart
Translation Chart of LIMS/SM
    Terms and Lab Terms
Users Chart
User-Event Routines Chart

These charts demonstrate that the amount of information used and managed by the LIMS is extensive. As much information about the system as possible should be gained in advance of installation and setup. (Of course, any of these parameters can be updated after installation and modified on-line.) Time spent on preinstallation planning is well spent. Installing a LIMS and creating a healthy LIMS environment is not an easy task, as discussed in Chapter 15. It is very important to the success of the project to begin with as much preparation as possible.

Security

Perhaps the most important setup parameters deal with security. There are two main aspects of security which must be defined during setup. One deals with user access to the LIMS itself and is controlled by the use of user IDs and passwords; the other deals with access to particular LIMS functions by LIMS users. When LIMS packages are installed and operated on multiuser, timesharing computer systems, protection of the LIMS from unauthorized use is very important. On such systems, the LIMS database can easily contain the most sensitive data in the system. This sensitivity is implanted by the strict requirement to guarantee integrity of the data. The LIMS must prevent unauthorized modifications to the data, whether inadvertent, malicious, or changes made by someone without proper authority.

Access to the LIMS

Many LIMS packages are expected to run on timesharing minicomputers which also host many other applications in addition to the LIMS. Typical access to this type of computer is guarded by a first-level user ID and password combination. The users of a large minicomputer include individuals who use only the LIMS, others who never use the LIMS, and still others who use the LIMS and other applications as well. In fact, one benefit of placing a LIMS on a large, general-purpose computer system as opposed to a dedicated LIMS computer is the availability of other software to LIMS users. Also, using LIMS data with statistical packages, word processors, spreadsheets, and user-written programs is simplified when everything is done on the same computer system. The use of a dedicated LIMS computer does have a slight advantage when it comes to security. The number of user accounts is certainly less and is easier to manage. When the dedicated LIMS computer is included on a local area network with other general purpose systems, the advantages of software availability, mentioned above, are slight.

Consideration of security should not preclude the installation of a LIMS on a large multiuser computer system. The advantages of running the LIMS on a large system outweigh the advantages of using a system dedicated only to the LIMS. Other considerations, such as price/performance, cost of maintenance, total number of users on the system, cost of hardware upgrades over time, etc., should be the criteria used to select the computer platform. Most of today's timesharing operating systems have the capability to control user access to programs and databases. For example, the DEC VAX/VMS operating system has several user access-related security levels, such as user ID and password, directory protection, file protection, and record protection. Access to any particular program or data file can either be granted or denied to any individual(s).

Maintaining control over user access is possible, but the importance of having this control is easily forgotten. The problems associated with maintaining user access control are not technological but procedural. LIMS management must include security considerations and user access control procedures which are part of everyday management. The time to begin user access control over a LIMS is during installation and setup. User accounts, disk directories, programs, data files, and databases must be set up to provide access only to a limited, known set of users. At one extreme, the LIMS manager and most of the LIMS support team must have total read-write-delete access to almost everything. At the other extreme, no account should have unrestricted access to particular areas, such as test results and revision histories.

Access to LIMS Functions

Once a LIMS user is granted access to the LIMS through a user ID and password, the set of functions available to the user must be controlled. Most LIMS packages have the capability to define which set of functions are available to each user. In some cases, functions may be defined, and then granted to users as sets instead of individually. For example, a sample submitter needs to have access to the following set of functions: (1) sample LOGIN, (2) cancel sample, (3) obtain sample status, and (4) view/print test results. There are other functions to which a submitter may be granted access, but there are some functions that would be withheld. A sample submitter would not be given access to functions that would be given to a lab analyst responsible for certain physical or analytical tests. These functions include: (1) enter and edit test results, (2) receive samples, (3) review test results, and (4) release test results. Each of these functions can be predefined during setup and granted as sets when new users are being defined.

LIMS users are presented with menus from which they select functions. A LIMS should be written such that only the functions available to a particular user appear on that user's menus. Several commercial LIMS packages operate in this manner. A major part of LIMS setup involves defining which functions will be available to different users. It is better to grant too few access privileges initially, and add necessary ones later, than to give too much access at the beginning.

Summary

The purchase of a LIMS is similar, in one way, to purchasing toys for a child. Toys come with the three words most feared by any parent: "Some assembly required." How many of us have uncovered this dreaded message, either late on Christmas Eve or on the night before a birthday party, and ended up working past midnight? The LIMS should be delivered with the same phrase highlighted on the outside of the package. LIMS setup is the preassembly necessary before the system can be used. Setting up is not complicated, but, it does require extensive planning. Better planning results in easier and more effective setup.

Practically every aspect of the LIMS/laboratory environment will need to be examined and then defined to the LIMS. We've noted that LIMS provides the opportunity to manage all information in a laboratory environment, and in doing so constitutes a new application technology. It should thus come as no surprise that before all this information can be managed with a computer system, it must be available to the system. Setup tasks are the methods used to transfer information about the lab environment to the LIMS.

Chapter 10

LIMS Supervisory Functions

Much of the functionality that is expected from a LIMS is not directly related to functions used for sample submission and testing or for test results storage and reporting. These additional functions are more closely related to extracting data from the system about the system — about samples and other lab-related items such as instruments, analysts, and tests. Table 10-1 provides a list of functionality which can be obtained using the LIMS supervisory functions. These supervisory functions can be used by managers to manage their laboratories. Day-to-day laboratory operations can be monitored, charted, and even predicted.

Raw data, component test results, calculated result values, and numerous associated times-of-day and dates are managed by a LIMS. In fact, these data will comprise most of the LIMS database. By having these data in a database, query techniques can be used to assimilate additional information about the data themselves. The LIMS supervisory functions provide this database access, and in doing so provide management tools for those who interact with the system.

The term *supervisory* is not intended to suggest that these functions are only for use by laboratory supervisors. The supervisory functions may be billed as tools for management, but this means that they are tools for managing. Every lab member must manage her or his job. The supervisory functions can help manage many aspects of a lab's business. The term supervisory is used to indicate that these functions operate at a level above some of the other LIMS functions. Figure 10-1 presents the level concept, illustrating the LIMS database as the lowest level, some of the more basic LIMS functions at the next level, and then two levels of supervisory functions. A more detailed evaluation of how the functions work together may yield even more levels.

As described in Chapter 3, a component of laboratory information management is data management. The supervisory functions begin where data management stops. Data management includes entering sample data in the database and possibly producing a results report.

Table 10-1. Functionality Provided by LIMS Supervisory Functions

---

1. scheduling
    — people
    — equipment
    — tests
    — samples
2. archive/restore
3. directories
    — tests
    — samples
    — sample types
    — customers
    — projects
    — instruments
4. reports
    — sample backlog
    — test backlog
    — control
    — cost invoice
    — device
    — exception
    — audit
    — status
    — trend

To a sample submitter, the quality of the result and the turnaround time for the analysis are the two primary concerns. Submitters want accurate answers, within acceptable limits, as quickly as possible. For the analytical laboratory manager to provide these responses, many details of the lab's operation must be managed. For example, large backlogs can be directly related to slow turnaround times.

When trying to decrease turnaround time, backlog management is a good place to begin. A good way to reduce the backlog is by efficient sample and resource scheduling. Before scheduling efficiency can be improved, however, measures must be devised by which levels of performance can be judged. Without such measures, there is no way to assess improvement. The supervisory functions can automatically provide the necessary measures on which to build management systems and improvement projects.

Supervisory Function Descriptions

Figure 10-2 lists some of the supervisory functions offered by the various LIMS packages. Some of these functions are described below.

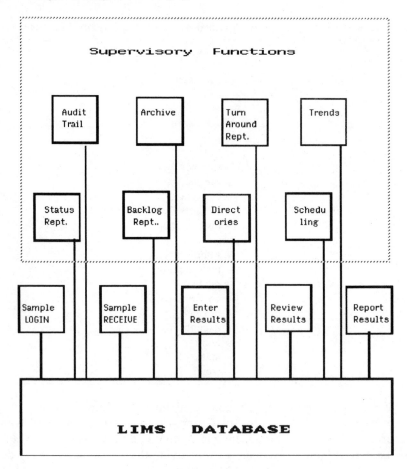

Figure 10-1. LIMS level concept.

Archive Function

The archive function removes sample information from the LIMS database and places it in a permanent storage medium. Accompanying the archive function is the retrieve function. Retrieval is not listed here as a separate function because it is understood that it must accompany an archive function.

Archive should not be confused with *backup*. Backup is a function performed on every computer system (hopefully) for two reasons: (1) to guard against inadvertent deletion of files, and (2) to guard against catastrophic failure of the system and/or disk drive(s). Backup of the LIMS should be done for these same reasons. The backup procedures maintained on the LIMS host may be sufficient for the LIMS itself, or the LIMS may include separate but similar procedures. Either way, backup

	AXIOM	BECKMAN	LIDMESC/SM	LAHBPSAM	NERPLLESAOBN	2P0E00	NAECPLCESEOSNS	VLAIRMISA/NDM	MAVNGAGER
Archive	X	X	X	X	X	X	X	X	X
Audit Trail Report	X	X	X	X		X	X	X	X
Backlog Report	X	X	X	X	X	X	X	X	X
Control Report	X	X	X	X			X	X	
Device Report		X	X	X		X	X	X	X
Directory Lists	X	X	X	X		X	X	X	X
Status Report	X	X	X	X	X	X	X	X	X
Trend Report	X	X	X			X	X	X	X
Turnaround Report	X		X	X		X	X	X	X

Figure 10-2. LIMS comparison — supervisory functions.

must be done for the LIMS daily. LIMS backup is not a supervisory function; it is a basic function which cannot be considered optional.

The purpose of the LIMS archive is to remove data from the database because the database size is not limitless and disk capacity is not cheap. But the archive function is not as simple as copying selected data from the database and thus freeing the database space for other entries. The system must also maintain permanent records of where and when individual samples were archived. The names of archive volumes, the associated date of the archive, and the sample IDs on the archive volume must be maintained.

The archive concept also indicates that the data are to be securely maintained for a long time, perhaps forever. The need to maintain archived data is not debatable. However, the practicality and feasibility of maintaining the data for long periods of time on a magnetic computer storage medium should be questioned. The accepted long-term storage medium is and has long been nine-track magnetic tape. But dependence on even this method is questionable, not because of the shelf life of the tape or the data stored on it, but owing to the rapidly changing computer industry. It is very likely that a computer tape created 20 years ago cannot be read today. Storage densities, operating systems, and tape file formats have all changed dramatically. The changes over the next 20 years will be even more dramatic. It will not be possible to use a removable disk for long term storage because even if the data did survive, it would be impractical and probably impossible to maintain a disk drive for 20 years. Disk drives may not even exist in the year 2010. LIMS archive procedures will change with time to accommodate new technologies. Even if nine-track tape remains the best long term storage medium, there is no guarantee that the LIMS will always read archived data the same way.

For these reasons, the archive function must continuously be given careful consideration. It may be necessary to convert all archived data from one format to another at certain times. For example, if a lab is maintaining archived data on 800 bpi tapes and the 800 bpi tape drive needs to be replaced, it is not practical to purchase another 800 bpi drive just to have compatibility with the old tapes. The tapes will have to be converted to the higher density of the new drive. Copying tapes every few years is not a bad idea anyway because tape does have a finite shelf life.

Audit Report

It is not accurate to say that any supervisory function is more important than others because every lab has different dependencies and different problems. However, the ability to guarantee the integrity of a result once it has been entered into the database is of primary importance to many laboratories, and perhaps should be to all. Thus, a major expectation of a LIMS is to provide a revision history and audit trail for sample test results and any other time-critical data. This feature seems to be gaining attention and importance as more and more labs realize the benefit of attaining paperless operations. Also, lab operating standards, whether in a government regulated environment or not, demand this type of security.

The audit trail capability does not merely mean having a report program to run when an audit trail report is needed. The backlog report function, for example, uses existing database entries for time, date, test and sample status to calculate the backlog. The database design is not altered to provide backlog capability. Providing audit trail capability, however, is a different story. The system and the database must be designed and operated in a particular manner to provide this capability. The ability to maintain an audit trail for every entry in the LIMS database is not a trivial task and it is not achieved without cost. Development times for in-house built systems are certainly affected when the audit capability is required. The cost of commercial systems is definitely increased by this capability. System performance is affected by making the user answer questions to indicate the reason for changing data items. Disk I/O is increased by reading and writing revision history records, which increase response time. Database size is increased, requiring more disk space, and thus increasing the cost of the computer system.

It is the combination of the audit trail design and database capability together with the audit report program that makes up the audit trail supervisory function. This function is probably the most complicated and possibly the most important LIMS function. It should certainly be included in any list of standard or core LIMS functions.

Figure 10-3 shows one type of audit report. This report contains every bit of information in the database related to the sample "P-ASH-RM10." Other reports can be structured to provide summary data on samples related to projects or batches, but it is important to be able to obtain easily all the information in the database about a sample.

Backlog Report

A backlog report contains information about a laboratory's outstanding test requests. This report is usually obtained as a printout, and some LIMS offer it in graphic form as well. Figure 10-4 shows the last page of a backlog report for the test code "GC-HYDROC." The sample information contained on the report includes worksheet ID, sample type, sample ID, aliquot ID, run number, date due, priority, and status. The summary at the end of the report shows 53 test requests with IL (In Lab) status, 39 with LG (Logged) status, and 82 with UT (Under Test) status. This type of data is valuable to the analyst responsible for the particular test and to the lab manager responsible for all tests. A sample log maintained manually as samples enter the lab could not account for samples with the LG status, because these are not yet in the lab.

A backlog report for a particular set of test codes can be scheduled to print in the laboratory responsible for those tests at preselected times, such as at the beginning of each shift. Analysts can then quickly see the workload distribution and begin planning to process the samples.

Control Report

A control report shows the test results for control samples. Control samples are used regularly to monitor the performance of testing procedures and instruments. Plotting results for control samples, maintaining test precision within a set of limits, and assigning a cause and correcting the reason for any points outside the limits are all part of instrument and sample management. Control reports can be numerical; however, the use of graphs usually makes it easier to spot trends.

```
        AUDIT REPORT                           3-DEC-1988
-------------------------------------------------------------------------- --

PRO_PROJECT_ID:                      LIMSTEST
CPJ_CLIENT_ID:                       LIMSMAN
SUB_SUBJECT_ID:                      LIMSMAN
SUB_CHANGE_DATE:                     1-DEC-1988 20:59:16.03
SUB_CHANGE_OPERATOR:                 LIMS System Manager
SUB_SUBJECT_NAME:                    TEST OF LIMS MODIFICATIONS
SUB_SUBJECT_TYPE:                    TEST
SUB_SUBJECT_LOCATION:                AS09 ADMIN SERVICES MANAGEMENT OF IC
SUB_COMMENTS: This is a dummy source for testing modifications to LIMS.
              These data can be archived to the bit bucket.
SUB_DESCRIPTOR_NAME:
SUB_DESCRIPTOR:
SAM_SAMPLE_ID:                       P-ASH-RM10
SAM_CHANGE_DATE:                     1-DEC-1988 15:28:01.27
SAM_CHANGE_OPERATOR:                 LIMS System Manager
SAM_SAMPLE_TYPE:                     MISC
SAM_REQUISITION_NUMBER:
SAM_SAMPLE_STATUS:                   RV
SAM_DEFAULT_TEST_LIMITS_TYPE:        NORMAL
SAM_COLLECTOR_ID:
SAM_LOGIN_OPERATOR_ID:               LIMS System Manager
SAM_RECEIPT_OPERATOR_ID:             LIMS System Manager
SAM_DATE_LOGGED:                     22-NOV-1988 18:10:15.28
SAM_DATE_DRAWN:                      22-NOV-1988 18:10:15.28
SAM_DATE_RECEIVED:                   22-NOV-1988 18:10:15.28
SAM_ACCOUNT_NUMBER:                  TEST
SAM_RETENTION_DATE:                  21-MAY-1989 18:10:15
SAM_DATE_COMPLETED:                  22-NOV-1988 18:38:43.42
SAM_DATE_REVIEWED:                   1-DEC-1988 15:28:01.27
SAM_DATE_APPROVED:
SAM_COMMENTS:
SAM_DESCRIPTOR_NAME:
TRL_COMPONENT_CODE:                  CRUC_TYPE
TRL_CHANGE_DATE:                     22-NOV-1988 18:12:42.03
TRL_CHANGE_OPERATOR:                 LIMS System Manager
TRL_TEST_RESULT:                     PORCELAIN
TRL_RESULT_FLAG:
TRL_COMPONENT_CODE:                  %ASH
TRL_CHANGE_DATE:                     22-NOV-1988 18:12:42.03
TRL_CHANGE_OPERATOR:                 LIMS System Manager
TRL_TEST_RESULT:                        40.00
TRL_RESULT_FLAG:
TRL_COMPONENT_CODE:                  NO_CYCLES
TRL_CHANGE_DATE:                     22-NOV-1988 18:12:42.03
TRL_CHANGE_OPERATOR:                 LIMS System Manager
TRL_TEST_RESULT:                     2
TRL_RESULT_FLAG:
TRL_COMPONENT_CODE:                  ASH_TYPE
TRL_CHANGE_DATE:                     22-NOV-1988 18:12:42.03
TRL_CHANGE_OPERATOR:                 LIMS System Manager
TRL_TEST_RESULT:                     OXIDE
TRL_RESULT_FLAG:
TRL_COMPONENT_CODE:                  TEMP
TRL_CHANGE_DATE:                     22-NOV-1988 18:12:42.03
TRL_CHANGE_OPERATOR:                 LIMS System Manager
TRL_TEST_RESULT:                     600
TRL_RESULT_FLAG:
```

Figure 10-3. Audit report — every data item for one sample.

```
TRL_COMPONENT_CODE:              TARE_WGT
TRL_CHANGE_DATE:                 22-NOV-1988 18:12:42.03
TRL_CHANGE_OPERATOR:             LIMS System Manager
TRL_TEST_RESULT:                 25.0
TRL_RESULT_FLAG:
TRL_COMPONENT_CODE:              FINAL_WGT
TRL_CHANGE_DATE:                 22-NOV-1988 18:12:42.03
TRL_CHANGE_OPERATOR:             LIMS System Manager
TRL_TEST_RESULT:                 27.0
TRL_RESULT_FLAG:
TRL_COMPONENT_CODE:              GROSS_WGT
TRL_CHANGE_DATE:                 22-NOV-1988 18:12:42.03
TRL_CHANGE_OPERATOR:             LIMS System Manager
TRL_TEST_RESULT:                 30.0
TRL_RESULT_FLAG:
TRQ_TEST_CODE:                   ASH
TRQ_TEST_LIMITS_TYPE:            NORMAL
TRQ_WORKSHEET_SEQ_NUMBER:        0
TRQ_CHANGE_DATE:                 1-DEC-1988 15:21:22.70
TRQ_CHANGE_OPERATOR:             CARL G KEARNEY
TRQ_TEST_STATUS:                 RA
TRQ_TOP_TEST_GROUP:
TRQ_MIDDLE_TEST_GROUP:
TRQ_DATE_RESULT_ENTERED:         22-NOV-1988 18:12:42.03
TRQ_DATE_RESULT_EDITED:
TRQ_DATE_RESULT_REVIEWED:        1-DEC-1988 15:21:22.70
TRQ_RAW_DATA_LOCATION:
TRQ_DEVICE_ID:
TRQ_TEST_OPERATOR_ID:            LIMS System Manager
TRQ_REVIEW_OPERATOR_ID:          CARL G KEARNEY
TRQ_PRIORITY:                    3
TRQ_RUN_NUMBER:                  1
ALI_ALIQUOT_ID:                  P
ALI_CHANGE_DATE:                 1-DEC-1988 15:28:01.11
ALI_CHANGE_OPERATOR:             LIMS System Manager
ALI_PRIORITY:                    3
ALI_ALIQUOT_LOCATION:
ALI_ALIQUOT_STATUS:              RV
ALI_DATE_SPLIT:                  22-NOV-1988 18:10:15.28
ALI_DATE_DUE:                    2-DEC-1988 18:10:15
ALI_DATE_COMPLETED:              22-NOV-1988 18:38:43.37
ALI_PARENT:
ALI_GRANDPARENT:
ALI_WORKSHEET_LOCATOR:
              ********** END OF REPORT **********
```

Figure 10-3 (*continued*)

A control report allows the results for control samples to be viewed separately from those of other samples. This separation is more useful when many instruments are involved.

Device Report

The device report lists the instrument types and the devices within each type which are known to the LIMS. Maintenance and circulation of the device report is a necessary form of communication between a lab and its customers. The instrument data are, of course, maintained by the lab. The device report can be printed and circulated to customers, or it can be accessed by the customer at any time on-line.

Test Backlog Report

Test Code: GC-HYDROC

Submitter Name	Sample Type	Sample ID	Run No.	Date Logged	Date Due	Status
RANDALL SIMMONS	MISC	15964301-01AMV	1	2-Dec-88	12-DEC-88	UT
RANDALL SIMMONS	MISC	15962301-01AMV	1	2-Dec-88	12-DEC-88	UT
RANDALL SIMMONS	MISC	15956801-01AMV	1	2-Dec-88	12-DEC-88	UT
RANDALL SIMMONS	MISC	15962401-01AMV	1	2-Dec-88	12-DEC-88	UT
TERRIE BAKER	MISC	X20605-043-11	1	1-Dec-88	11-DEC-88	UT
TERRIE BAKER	MISC	X20605-043-1	1	1-Dec-88	11-DEC-88	UT
TERRIE BAKER	MISC	X20605-043-12	1	1-Dec-88	11-DEC-88	UT
TERRIE BAKER	MISC	X20605-043-2	1	1-Dec-88	11-DEC-88	UT
TERRIE BAKER	MISC	X20605-042-1	1	1-Dec-88	11-DEC-88	UT
TERRIE BAKER	MISC	X20605-042-10	1	1-Dec-88	11-DEC-88	UT
TERRIE BAKER	MISC	X20605-042-2	1	1-Dec-88	11-DEC-88	UT
TERRIE BAKER	MISC	X20605-043-3	1	1-Dec-88	11-DEC-88	UT
TERRIE BAKER	MISC	X20605-042-11	1	2-Dec-88	12-DEC-88	UT
TERRIE BAKER	MISC	X20605-042-3	1	2-Dec-88	12-DEC-88	UT
TERRIE BAKER	MISC	X20605-043-4	1	2-Dec-88	12-DEC-88	UT
TERRIE BAKER	MISC	X20605-042-12	1	2-Dec-88	12-DEC-88	UT
TERRIE BAKER	MISC	X20605-042-4	1	2-Dec-88	12-DEC-88	UT
TERRIE BAKER	MISC	X20605-043-5	1	2-Dec-88	12-DEC-88	UT
TERRIE BAKER	MISC	X20605-042-5	1	2-Dec-88	12-DEC-88	UT
TERRIE BAKER	MISC	X20605-043-6	1	2-Dec-88	12-DEC-88	UT
TERRIE BAKER	MISC	X20605-042-6	1	2-Dec-88	12-DEC-88	UT
TERRIE BAKER	MISC	X20605-043-7	1	2-Dec-88	12-DEC-88	UT
TERRIE BAKER	MISC	X20605-042-7	1	2-Dec-88	12-DEC-88	UT
TERRIE BAKER	MISC	X20605-043-8	1	2-Dec-88	12-DEC-88	UT
TERRIE BAKER	MISC	X20605-042-8	1	2-Dec-88	12-DEC-88	UT
TERRIE BAKER	MISC	X20605-043-9	1	2-Dec-88	12-DEC-88	UT
TERRIE BAKER	MISC	X20605-042-9	1	2-Dec-88	12-DEC-88	UT
TERRIE BAKER	MISC	X20605-043-10	1	2-Dec-88	12-DEC-88	UT
BARRY OLIVER	MISC	X20528-136	1	2-Dec-88	12-DEC-88	UT
BARRY OLIVER	MISC	X20528-137	1	2-Dec-88	12-DEC-88	UT
BARRY OLIVER	MISC	X20528-138	1	2-Dec-88	12-DEC-88	UT
MARY E. BOONE	MISC	X17709-143A-1	1	2-Dec-88	12-DEC-88	UT
MARY E. BOONE	MISC	X17709-143A-2	1	2-Dec-88	12-DEC-88	UT
MARY E. BOONE	MISC	X17709-143B-1	1	2-Dec-88	12-DEC-88	UT
MARY E. BOONE	MISC	X17709-143B-2	1	2-Dec-88	12-DEC-88	UT

Summary for Test Code GC-HYDROC   :

53 Test Requests with Status IL
39 Test Requests with Status LG
82 Test Requests with Status UT

174 Test Requests for Test Code GC-HYDRC

********** END OF REPORT *********

Figure 10-4. Backlog report.

Directory List

Lists of items which comprise the LIMS database, such as customers, projects, samples, sample types, and reports, can be referred to as *directory lists*. These lists are called different things by different LIMS such as *dictionary lists* or *catalog lists*. These lists are similar in concept to other lists, such as the list of instruments obtained by the device report. Directory lists are not reports but are more like help tools. For example, if a LIMS user is logging in a sample for a particular GC analysis but doesn't know the exact name of the test, a directory list of tests would be useful. The ability to access a directory list without canceling out of the LIMS function provides the highest level of utility for the directory function.

Status Report

The status report, sometimes called the *progress report,* is primarily used to obtain quickly the status and any completed results for a sample. This function is very useful for sample submitters who want to find out the status of their samples. Use of this function eliminates the need to call the testing lab. Thus, it is an important time saver.

Trend Report

The trend report is usually a graph which plots test results against time, thus providing the capability to see developing patterns or trends. When analyzing samples from sequential production batches, trend reports and analysis are very important. Trend reports, or graphs, are relatively simple to maintain manually, but this is time-consuming. By having the LIMS maintain the trend graph automatically, the time requirement is eliminated. Even more important, the chance for human error is eliminated. In addition, the graph can be automatically printed at selected intervals, thus eliminating all the human requirements for producing the graph.

Turnaround Report

The time between sample availability for analysis and production of the final report is known as the *turnaround time.* Turnaround time, in conjunction with the accuracy and precision of the test results, are two of the most important aspects of sample processing. This should be true from both the lab's and the customer's point of view.

It is sometimes hard to measure the effectiveness of a particular laboratory. Assume that an analytical laboratory has a turnaround time of 3 days for the majority of sample types analyzed. This turnaround time can be decreased by adding staff and instruments or by enhancing automation. We must answer the question, "What should the turnaround time be?" Perhaps 3 days is sufficient. There is only one way to answer this question: We must understand the customer's fitness-for-use crite-

```
                        Turnaround Time Report

Selection Criteria:
    Source ID: UL839380
    Sample Type: MISC
    Test Code: IV
    Date to Report on:   3-DEC-1988


                              Test Requests
                              -------------

               Current #  Mean Days  Mean Days    Percent in State X Days
    State      in State   in State   Since LG   0-5   6-10 11-15 16-20  >20
--------------  --------   --------   --------   -----  ----- ----- ----- ----
Logged    (LG):     8        1.0        1.0    100 %   0 %   0 %   0 %   0 %
In Lab    (IL):    44        2.5        2.5    100 %   0 %   0 %   0 %   0 %
Under Test(UT):    19        0.0        1.6    100 %   0 %   0 %   0 %   0 %
Complete  (CO):     0        0.0        0.0      0 %   0 %   0 %   0 %   0 %
                ========
       Total:      71


*************** END OF REPORT ****************
```

Figure 10-5. Turnaround time report.

rion for turnaround time. How quickly does the customer want the results? Even better, how quickly does the customer need the results? What factors determine the customer's expectations for turnaround time? Is it personnel scheduling, equipment scheduling, or control of a manufacturing process? It is very important for the lab to know the customer's expectations and the purpose of the results. If lab members know that a manufacturing process is controlled with the test results and that a 20 minute turnaround is expected, they will usually try their best to meet that deadline or even better it.

Determining a customer's expectations and fitness-for-use criterion is sometimes not easy. Many sample submitters want the test results as quickly as possible. They might say that they want a 3-day turnaround because that is what they have been getting and have come to expect. But when does sample turnaround genuinely affect the customer's business? At what point does the lack of a test result become an impediment to the customer? In many cases, the lab must assist its customers in answering these questions. However, before a customer can be approached concerning his or her turnaround time requirements, the lab must have its processes in control and must be able to prove it. Turnaround time measures are important indicators of how well a lab is performing.

There are probably as many different methods of calculating and reporting turnaround time as there are laboratories that measure it. Creative use of this measure can provide an effective tool when helping a customer determine fitness-for-use. Figure 10-5 shows a turnaround time report for a particular customer and test. Perhaps the ultimate use of these data would be to collect it daily, add selected points to a graph daily, and then print the graph weekly and send it to the customer — automatically by the LIMS, with no human intervention. When a lab can provide this type of information in a reliable and routine manner, the lab establishes a point of reference for all negotiations and interactions with the customer. The customer might be willing to pay for more personnel and/or instruments to reduce the turnaround time, but not if the lab is perceived to be inefficient and unresponsive. Of course, merely giving turnaround time information to the customer doesn't mean that the lab is operating in a controlled, efficient manner. But if it is, this type of information can document its performance.

Summary

To process a sample in a laboratory using a LIMS requires the use of a set of functions which we have called the standard, or core, functions. Supervisory functions differ from standard functions in that they are not needed to process a sample. They provide data about the system and its components in order to plan for and subsequently improve lab processes.

The supervisory functions are a combination of functions and features, some complex and others relatively simple. We can probably consider several of the supervisory functions as standard. They are required for continued efficient use of the LIMS and are offered in various forms by the commercial products. In some ways, the supervisory functions mark the difference between a data management system and a LIMS.

For those laboratories in the process of installing a LIMS, imaginative use of the supervisory functions can mean the difference between making lab members use the new system and giving them tools to help them do their jobs better.

Chapter 11

Managing a LIMS

In previous chapters, we have examined many aspects of laboratories and the management of information related to sample processing. We have looked at the use of LIMS packages as tools with which to gather, interpret, report, store, and provide audit trails for test results and to manage all types of laboratory information. We have seen that efficiency increases as a result of laboratory automation and that LIMS can be used as a backbone for automation projects. However, to this point, we have not investigated the factors in determining LIMS requirements, evaluating methods of obtaining a LIMS, installation, operation, or support of a LIMS.

The management of a LIMS is not just the day-to-day operation of the system once it is in place; the process begins much sooner. It involves a great deal of preliminary work in specifying requirements and selecting or writing a system. Just as important, for a LIMS to be successful, the LIMS manager must be involved daily in "selling" the system to lab management and LIMS users. There has to be more user "buy-in" early in the implementation phase, but widespread acceptance within the laboratory will be slow.

Factors that influence LIMS management are listed in Table 11-1 and examined in the following sections. After discussing some of the LIMS management concerns, we will see that the LIMS manager must have a certain combination of characteristics and skills in order to run the system effectively. This combination is examined in the Summary.

Factors That Influence LIMS Management

Size and Complexity of the LIMS

The size and complexity (scope) of the LIMS implementation will make a big difference in nearly all system management considerations. The size of an implementation cannot be measured by the number of samples

Table 11-1. Factors That Influence LIMS Management

I. Size and complexity of the LIMS
II. Elements of change
   — Requirements change
   — New features need to be added
III. Determining system requirements, preselection planning
   — Define laboratories, tests, customers, instrumentation, data input and report output formats
IV. Selecting the LIMS software
   — Market survey
   — Write a LIMS in-house
     > Software development life cycle
     > Database selection
     > Code verification
     > Post installation support
   — Contract a LIMS
     > Hire contract programmer(s)
     > Hire firm specializing in LIMS contract programming
   — Purchase a LIMS from a vendor
     > Vendor presentations
     > Software demonstrations
V. The software system lifespan
   — Preinstallation planning
   — Installation
   — Learning for support personnel
   — Learning for users
   — Intense support
   — Continuing support
VI. Buy-in
   — Top-down support
   — Management overview

alone. A system with only a few test methods which handles 1000 samples per week is not as complex as a system with 100 test methods and 1000 samples per week. More test methods mean more raw data formats, whether collected from an instrument or entered from the keyboard. Generally, the size of a LIMS implementation is related to the number of samples processed, while its complexity is related to the number of tests methods. Differences in dependence on LIMS supervisory functions, sample tracking, and training also represent major differences in complexity.

Although complexity is hard to measure and is a relative term when dealing with a LIMS, size can certainly be quantified. The following table identifies LIMS systems as small, medium, large, or very large, based on the number of samples per week:

Size of the LIMS	Number of Samples per Week
Small	<200
Medium	200–1000
Large	1000–2000
Very Large	>2000

Obviously, more complex LIMS projects will require more management. Systems based on a single PC connected to one or two instruments are easy to set up and operate by one person who has other duties as well. Systems with dozens of test methods and connected to dozens of instruments require a full-time manager (24).

A large LIMS requires more hardware "horsepower" than a small LIMS. A large LIMS built on a large timesharing mini or supermini must share system resources with other applications. The LIMS will have to be managed in conjunction with management of the computer system itself. The LIMS manager and the system manager will be required to work hand-in-hand on a daily basis. System shutdowns by the system manager, for software installation or hardware reconfiguration need to be scheduled with the LIMS manager.

As described in Chapter 3, the use of PCs in the lab is common. As a result, the development of LIMS on PCs has also occurred (24). Small LIMS on dedicated PCs or minis require much less external coordination to operate. But even PCs require down time for maintenance, software installation and modification, and backup. When a dedicated PC is off-line for whatever reason, other related functions will likely be affected. But for PC based systems, these effects will certainly be less widespread, will involve fewer people, and will be much easier to schedule.

Elements of Change

Even the simplest computer program or system requires attention from time to time if its use is to continue. The more extensive the system, the more support it requires. As in a well-oiled machine, computer software parts fit together fine at first, but use spans time. What happens with time? Requirements change, causing parts not to fit as well as they once did. What else happens? Better parts become available. Hardware upgrades sometime require program modifications. Job assignments change. New people have new ideas. More economical or faster methods are designed and require program modifications. When more and more data are added, dimensions overrun requiring modifications. Support of software systems means understanding how they work and having the ability to make modifications as required. Thus, for any software system, modifications are required as time passes for two reasons:

1. Requirements change for existing features.
2. New features must be implemented.

Continued use of any software system requires a manager to see that necessary modifications get made. A system for which there is no manager, or no one responsible, dies early — or at best is underutilized (25). Continued use of a LIMS requires a manager to oversee day-to-day operations. In fact, the number of benefits derived from any LIMS installation is directly proportional to how well the system is managed; and LIMS managers change as assignments change, retirements occur, and promotions are earned. The most important function of any manager is to train his or her successor. This successor should come from within the LIMS support team.

The functional and physical life expectancy of computer hardware is increasing with each new model. It is currently from 5–10 years. Computers wear out and become unreliable and expensive to maintain. The increased performance of new models and the relatively high maintenance expense of older models can easily justify replacement — which is the source of another element of change.

Management of the above changes, and others, is critical to the success of any computer related system. The elements of change will subject the system to erosion, just as the elements of weather affect the Earth. Effort, expense, and capital will be required to survive the elements of change. The LIMS manager should be forewarned, and hopefully should be experienced, in dealing with computer systems in order to handle the inevitable changes.

Determining System Requirements: Preselection Planning

Preselection planning is a preliminary evaluation, done before considering possible software vendors or other LIMS sources, to determine the scope of the project. It is the first step in putting a LIMS in place. The results of the evaluation will be used either to custom design a LIMS or as system specifications to discuss with LIMS vendors as they demonstrate their products. The actual management of the LIMS begins with preselection planning. Thus, the LIMS manager must be named, in place, and responsible for all planning and subsequent installation.

To conduct the preselection planning, a team should be formed which we will call the preselection *analytical team,* led by the LIMS manager and consisting of representatives from each testing and customer lab, as well as anyone who will be involved in defining analytical specifications. Generally, the team should be considered a "natural" team, consisting of those who might use the LIMS once installed. Of course, the initial selection of team members will have to be a "best guess." As the responsibilities of the team are clarified, it will be become clearer who the members should be, and adjustments can be made. The analytical team should only be involved in gathering information from the analytical viewpoint. That is, this team should not consider any hardware- or software-related topics; only laboratory-related topics are their concern. Therefore, representatives (systems analysts) from the software development department, if available, would purposely be excluded from this team.

There are organizations which specialize in laboratory consulting (32) that can be employed by the analytical team when help is needed. Some of the services offered include feasibility studies, functional specification development, and laboratory surveys.

Table 11-2 summarizes the responsibilities of the analytical team, which are discussed below:

1. *Define the laboratories. The testing laboratories and areas within laboratories, where necessary, in which the LIMS is to be applied are identified. It is not desirable to include all lab areas under the LIMS umbrella. For example, a method development lab would typically be modifying methods so rapidly during the development stages that it would be a waste of effort to use LIMS for these methods. Also, this lab would not be analyzing many customer samples and thus would not benefit from using LIMS features.*
2. *Define the tests. The number of analytical tests to be managed by the LIMS must be determined. This determination should also include an identification of all test components for all tests. For example, each GC or LC method would be counted as a separate test. The retention*

Table 11-2. Responsibilities of the Preselection Analytical Team

Responsibilities of the Preselection Analytical Team
1. Define the analytical testing laboratories which will use the LIMS.
2. Define analytical tests to be managed by the LIMS.
3. Define number of samples to be processed per week.
4. Define the customers — those who will submit samples using the LIMS.
5. Define data "end-use" — how the data will ultimately be used.
6. Define the instrumentation which requires automated data entry into the LIMS.
7. Define nonstandard data input and report output formats.

times, peak areas, and calculated concentrations for each named peak would be separate test components. Other components are the internal standard ratio, sample weight, etc.

The analytical team may include some tests in the initial evaluation which will later be considered inappropriate. However, this is to be expected. The methods and tests to include will become more evident as the evaluation proceeds. The initial test and component counts are only estimates. It is better to estimate too many test components than too few. System requirements such as database size, CPU and memory sizes, etc., will be specified based on these findings.

3. **Define the number of samples.** The number of samples to be processed by the LIMS must be determined. The size of the LIMS implementation is proportional to the number of samples processed by the LIMS. Those implementing very large systems will have to pay close attention to any size limitations of vendor packages. Those with smaller systems can place more emphasis on other aspects of LIMS packages.

4. **Define the customers.** Once the set of testing laboratories and tests have been defined, the customers for those labs and tests must be identified. The customers are those who will use the LIMS to submit samples to the identified testing labs for the identified tests. We have stated that the analytical team may need to adjust its membership as it gathers more detailed information. As customers are identified, the team should make sure that they are represented.

5. **Define data end use.** An important aspect of a LIMS directly related to its benefit potential deals with how test result data are ultimately used. The LIMS must provide graphs for customers who want them; a variety of database searches for those who sometimes need to relate data differently; and statistics, archiving, and audit trails for others. The end use of the data managed by the LIMS must be defined.

6. **Define the instrumentation.** The instruments which will perform the tests to be managed by the LIMS must be identified. As described in Chapters 2, 3, and 7, automation of test results entry offers as much if not more benefit than any other form of lab automation. The pipelining of data from the instrument directly into the LIMS is the ideal method of data entry. For this reason, it is important to know all instruments which might be candidates for automated data collection. A list of these instruments will be needed during LIMS software selection (or development). The ability to interface the necessary instrumentation will likely be one of the determining factors in LIMS selection.

7. **Define nonstandard data input and report output formats.** Some laboratory tests require more data, from the submitter than others. These

data are typically supplied on a test-specific submission form which accompanies the sample to the laboratory. Identification of these special submission forms is important because inclusion of any extra data in a LIMS sample LOGIN process will most likely require modification or customization of the LIMS.

Sometimes a laboratory's customers demand that their reports be returned in a nonstandard format. It is important to identify nonstandard report requirements because they also will likely require modification or customization of the LIMS.

All of the definitions and determinations should be made for both current and projected future requirements. They should be specified as now, now $+2$ years, and now $+5$ years. These projections will play a major role in the selection of the LIMS.

Selecting the LIMS Software

Once the preselection analytical team has completed the requirements definition, a LIMS must be obtained. There are three ways to obtain LIMS software — write it, contract the job, or purchase a package from a LIMS vendor. Some laboratories have the ability to write their own LIMS; others do not. Hardware dependence or inclination, such as PC versus mainframe, will play a role in software selection. Some vendors offer LIMS packages for PC, mini, and mainframe computers; others offer-PC only packages, and still others offer mini and mainframe packages. Steps and considerations for selecting the LIMS software are discussed in the following sections.

Do Market Survey. A market survey of commercially available LIMS packages should be the next step. Vendors should be contacted, literature gathered, and product demonstrations set up. Laboratories with the ability to write their own LIMS may pick up many valuable new ideas about methodology or database design which could be built into their own systems, or, they may find a package which could be purchased and implemented for substantially less than the cost of in-house development. Thus, the logical next step after requirements definition for anyone considering a LIMS implementation is a market survey.

A new team, known as the *selection team,* should be assembled to conduct the market survey and select software. It should also be lead by the LIMS manager. The only difference between this team and the analytical team is that the selection team should include computer support people as well. Systems analysts familiar with the hardware and other software from the different LIMS vendors will be needed for detailed system scrutiny. Knowing what questions to ask during product demonstrations could easily identify a system which stands above the others in meeting a particular set of requirements. It is a good idea to rotate some new customer representatives into the new team. This will give more people the feeling that they have contributed to the development of the LIMS; this will pay off in needed support during installation and gearing up.

The market survey should be conducted with several system requirements in mind. These requirements, summarized in Table 11-3, are as follows:

1. *Proper size.* The LIMS should be big enough to encompass the expected number of:
   a. *Test methods and components.* Some LIMS databases are sized according to the total number of components. One test method may be composed of a dozen or more components. As mentioned above, a GC or LC method is composed of many components.
   b. *Samples.* The number of samples to be processed by the LIMS is the single most important sizing factor for database considerations.
   c. *Simultaneous users.* The estimate of the number of simultaneous users must be based on the number of estimated samples, sample submitters, and testing labs which will be using the LIMS. It will

Table 11-3. LIMS Requirements to be Evaluated During the Market Study

1. Proper size
2. Growth potential
3. Interface to instrumentations
4. Customizable data input
5. Customizable report output
6. Interface to user-written code
7. Support
   — Installation
   — Continuing
8. Hardware requirements
   — CPU and memory
   — Terminals
9. Ad hoc database access
10. Cost
    — Initial system cost
    — Continuing vendor support cost
    — In-house support cost
11. Ease of use

certainly be a best guess, but it is important enough to warrant considerable preliminary effort.

2. *Growth potential.* Growth in the LIMS environment for at least 5 years should be projected for the number of labs, samples, users, and instrumentation. A primary concern in selecting any software is how it will perform in a few years.

3. *Interface to the desired mix of instrumentation for automation of results entry.* Automation of results entry is the single best way to increase lab efficiency. Some LIMS packages interface readily to the same vendor's instruments. LIMS vendors should be asked to provide interfacing examples and assistance for any make or model of instrument. They should be presented with the list of instruments for which interfacing is desired and asked for specific recommendations on how they can be interfaced.

4. *Customizable data input formats.* Some tests require more preliminary information than others before they can be run. For example, a thermal analysis request form is illustrated in Figure 11-1. The sample submitter must mark the desired boxes indicating the analyses required. In order to include this test in a LIMS, the LIMS must be able to handle a customized form of this type. A separate test code could be defined for each test listed on the form, but that would not be desirable.

5. *Customizable data output formats.* It should be expected that about half of the sample submitters to a LIMS will want their results back in a nonstandard format. The analytical team will have defined some of these formats, but as LIMS users become more familiar with the system and its capabilities, they will start making requests for output in different forms. For example, they may request that results for a particular set of tests be automatically entered into a spreadsheet for subsequent statistical analyses.

6. *Interface to user-written code for customization.* The previously described customizable input and output formats will rely on user-written code for implementation. Although most LIMS do offer variable standard report formats, such as indicating which data items to include on the result report, more complex result manipulations will require user-written code.

    Some of the other functions requiring user-written code are instrument and computer interfacing, help screens, billing, interfacing to other software systems and databases, automated results reporting, and database search routines.

7. *Support*
    a. *Installation support.* The exact requirements for installation support should be presented to vendors during the market survey.

LIMS THERMAL ANALYSIS REQUEST

SAMPLE ID: X20653-27-1 ____   CROSSREFERENCE NUMBER _____

ALIQUOT_ID: P ___

ALIQUOT STATUS: LG

Analysis Required:

DTA: _ in N2   _ in air

TGA: _ in N2   _ in air
            _ scanning _ isothermal at _____ degrees C

TMA: _____ degrees C to _____ degrees C

DSC: Transitions to be determined:
                X Tg   X Tch   X Tm   X Tcc
                X heats of transition
                _ heatset temperature or other heat history

            Scans required:
                X first heating
                X second heating
                X cooling from melt

            Crystallization halftimes:
                (Please see OPTIONAL SPECIFICATIONS below)
                _ from melt
                _ from glass

            OPTIONAL SPECIFICATIONS:
            The maximum temperature to be used for melting is 160____ degrees C

            The temperature (or temperature ranges) to be used for
            halftime determinations are: _____ degrees C

            HELPFUL INFORMATION:
            The approx. Tg is (are): 0_____

COMMENTS:

Figure 11-1. Thermal analysis request form.

If these requirements are unclear, they should be discussed in detail and clarified with each vendor. LIMS installations are usually handled on an individual basis because each is different and presents unique problems and opportunities.

b. *Continuing support.* Various levels of support are available from most LIMS vendors. The type of support required should be discussed with each vendor. Vendor support options range from none to having a full-time resident on site. An attractive intermediate level consists of telephone hotline service plus upgrades and new versions of the LIMS when released.

8. *Hardware requirements*

   a. *CPU and memory.* The greater the requirement for the number of simultaneous users, the higher the CPU horsepower requirement. For any system larger than a single user PC, response time is a critical factor. Large CPUs with large main memories will be required for medium-sized to large LIMS packages in order to maintain adequate response time.

   b. *Terminal types.* Graphics, windows, and forms are (or are becoming) standard LIMS features, either as built-in functions or in conjunction with externally linked graphics/statistics packages. In many cases, these features are limited to specific types/brands of terminals. The terminal hardware requirements must be discussed with each vendor in detail, especially when the LIMS will be linked to external software.

9. *Ad hoc database access.* The ability to provide ad hoc database access from within the LIMS is a useful feature. For those who desire variations in data relationships, this feature, or some user-written database search code, is a requirement.

10. *Cost.*

    a. *Initial system, including installation.* The initial cost of the system, like that of most other software products, will likely be related to CPU size or the number of simultaneous users. For some packages, installation is optional. For others, it is included in the purchase price. The installation price must be discussed with each vendor.

    b. *Continuing vendor support.* The cost of continuing vendor support on a yearly basis should be not be neglected. It will be about 10-15% of the selling price for a telephone hotline plus new-release support.

    c. *In-house support.* The cost, or fractional cost, of the LIMS manager and any other LIMS support personnel must be estimated. Each vendor should be asked to help with this estimate after gaining a knowledge of the system's requirements. There will be a minimum support level below which the project will not survive. Generally, the benefit level is proportional to the support level. It will be possible to determine an optimum support level after gaining experience with the system.

11. *Ease of use.* Most LIMS are designed to be easy to use. In many instances, first-time LIMS users, from scientist to plant operator, may also be using a computer for the first time as well. Hands-on demonstrations are required in order to evaluate ease of use. A

vendor, understandably, is so familiar with the product that its use looks simple. Let the vendors assist members of the selection team to use the LIMS during presentations.

The above system requirements are not listed in any particular order. Their relative importance will vary from installation to installation. For example, if a large minicomputer is already available to use as the LIMS host, the hardware requirement will be less important during vendor meetings. Also, the ad hoc database access will be less important if no customers were identified who need it or if user-written code can provide variable data searches.

When the market survey is complete, the selection team must decide how to obtain the LIMS software. It is not likely that one system will meet all the requirements exactly. One of the following scenarios is more likely to be the result of the survey:

One system was identified which meets more of the requirements than other systems.

Two or more systems were seen which might work equally well.

No system stood out more than any other; all were about the same.

At this point, some organizations will be faced with the decision of either purchasing a LIMS package or writing their own. The following section describes the concerns associated with writing a LIMS in-house. As we will see, writing a medium-sized or large LIMS is a monumental undertaking. It would be lengthy and expensive, and would require a system development team project.

Write a LIMS In House.   The size and complexity of the LIMS to be written are the most significant factors in determining the ultimate complexity of the development project. Small systems can be written by small teams. For large systems to be implemented in an acceptable time frame, large development teams are required. For discussion purposes, we will assume the need to develop a medium-sized or large, fairly complex LIMS. Some critical factors to be considered before and during system development are summarized in Table 11-4 and discussed in the following sections.

Table 11-4. Critical Factors for Writing a LIMS

1. Software development life cycle
2. Database selection
3. Code verification
4. Post-installation support

1. *Software development life cycle*. For the most part, a LIMS can be developed using the same approach used to development any software system. Laboratory personnel, especially those on the selection team, and laboratory management should be made aware of this very complex, lengthy, and highly regimented procedure. The software development life cycle is illustrated in Figure 11-2. Although only the requirements analysis step is partially broken down into its components, this gives a good indication of the complexity of the development process. Writing a complicated software system is not just a matter of having a few programmers write code. Extensive planning, designing, and documenting accompany every line of code written. The actual coding of the programs is only a small part of the overall project.

   A third team should be created to function during software development. We will call this team the *development team*. It too should be led by the LIMS manager and should consist of the members of the selection team plus those systems analysts and programmers who will do the development. As suggested above, some new members from the laboratory might be rotated into the team as a means of providing a more widespread knowledge of the LIMS. A significant amount of time (10-20%) should be allowed for each laboratory team member to confer with the program developers. The time commitment of this team is a cost which should not be forgotten when considering in-house development costs.

   The LIMS manager will be required to work with the developers on a full-time basis. The requirements specified by the analytical team will have to be translated into program functions and code. The LIMS manager and the other laboratory members of the team must make sure that all requirement specifications are completely understood and not leave anything to chance or a programmer's best guess.

   Again, depending on the size and complexity of the LIMS, development times of many months should be expected. Use of new 4GL development tools can dramatically decrease development times (20). Other techniques, such as staging the development process, can be used to implement parts of the system as they are developed. For example, sample LOGIN and RESULTS REPORT could be the first functions written, tested, installed, and used. Staging development in this manner requires much up-front planning and coordination by all members of the team. Before bringing a new function on-line, training must be completed for the initial users. Other decisions, such as how long to operate the old and new systems simultaneously, must be made by the team in advance.

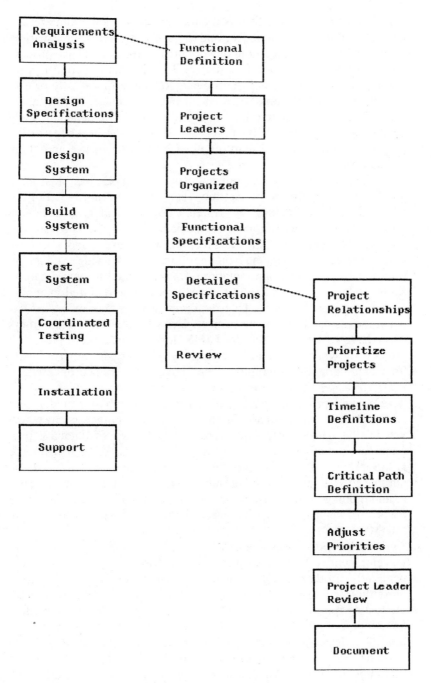

Figure 11-2. Software development life cycle.

2. *Database selection.* A LIMS is a database application. Data are collected, stored in the database, and subsequently used for a variety of purposes. During the initial development steps, a database product must be chosen on which to build the LIMS. This selection is very important to the success of the project. Response times, ease of use, growth, search functions (such as ad hoc searching), maintenance, ease of modification, and other important features will depend heavily on the database software itself. The database is the backbone of the LIMS. All functions and features must be written to use and share the database.

It's been a slow process, but database technology has blossomed and begun to mature in the last few years. Many, if not most, of the applications being written by systems development groups can be termed *database applications.* A specialized group of software developers has emerged, known as *database analysts* and *database programmers.* The demands on their time are growing, and many traditional language programmers are being trained in new database skills. Database analysts and programmers will be required members of the development team. This requirement places an increased expense or justification on the project. Even if database programmers don't have to be hired for the LIMS development, there are other projects on which they won't be working. Or there are other projects for which database programmers will have to be trained or hired.

Database selection is the single most important part of the LIMS development process. Ideally, there will be a database product with all the right features already in place on the computer system which will be the LIMS host. And there will be a host of database programmers already familiar with the product to be scheduled for the LIMS project. If this is not the case, a database will have to be purchased. The cost of buying the database software, learning to use it, and training the database programmers must not be forgotten. These costs must be included when considering whether to purchase or write a LIMS.

3. *Code verification.* As program modules are developed, they are tested. Development testing techniques call first for testing a module independently of other modules whenever possible. This technique allows more thorough testing because less code is involved. Integrated module testing follows as more modules are developed. Maintaining documentation of all testing is crucial to validation of the system. Every line of code must be tested. Every branch, GOTO, and IF-THEN must be executed, with documentation of the results.

Computer systems validation requires code validation during development. If the LIMS is not intended for resale or for a regulated environment, the developer might be tempted to slight code verification. But as we will state in Chapter 14, every computer system developed and/or operated must be required to conform to a validation protocol which guarantees that the system is performing as expected.

Testing software is always easier when it is being written, compared to later when the programmer is working on something else. Code verification should always be treated as a requirement, never as an option. Proper development techniques include verification as a means of quality assurance. A successful LIMS will not be achieved without the dedication to development of the highest quality software.

4. *Post installation support.* Post installation support of any large software system requires personnel dedicated to the task. This type of support mainly includes making the modifications required by changes, as described above. Whether a LIMS is purchased or written in-house, a *support team* will have to be established. Continuing support and the support team are discussed below in the section on "Computer Software System Life Span."

The support team must consist of the LIMS manager, a lab member(s) familiar with the laboratory operation, and a member(s) familiar with the system. Furthermore, it is desirable to include one of the system's developers on the support team. A primary objective of this person will be to train other programmers in how to modify the system so that as team members change, support will continue. Modifying an in-house written system may actually be easier than for a purchased system because all the source code will be available. More extensive modifications will be possible as time passes. Support of in-house written systems is often inadequate. As long as one or more of the original programmers has, or shares, responsibility for support, use of the system will continue without too many problems. In addition, new features, bug fixes, and design changes will still be implemented. But after a period of time, the original programmers move on to other projects. Without continued maintenance, the system will no longer meet all the requirements because these requirements change, as described above in the section on "Elements of Change." Without someone to make the necessary modifications over time, the system will not survive.

Obviously, the single programmer approach to developing anything more than a small LIMS is not appropriate. Development and support must be done by a team if the system is to survive in the long run. Corners cannot be cut in either development or support. The functionality of the final system depends on database selection. If an inadequate database is selected, the system will not expand in the future. Code verification is lengthy and expensive, but it must be done. Code verification is an integral part of a properly designed computer system validation protocol for a LIMS.

Contract a LIMS. For a laboratory writing its own LIMS, contract programmers can be added to the development staff to decrease the development time. The main requirement for these programmers might be experience with the hardware and the programming language being used. Contract programmers can be found to design and implement instrument-to-computer/LIMS connections. The requirement specification for this type of work would obviously be more stringent than for an assistant programmer.

Contracting the entire LIMS project is another option. It was mentioned above, in conjunction with defining specifications for the LIMS project, that certain organizations specialize in laboratory consulting. These same organizations (32) also offer customized LIMS installations. However, even if contracting the LIMS is the chosen solution, there must still be a team to manage the project. The team is responsible for defining the system specifications, defining project milestones and target dates, working with the contractors on a daily basis, and testing modules to make sure that the specifications are being met. The team must be committed to support the system after completion. The system cannot just be installed and forgotten. Computer software is like a machine. If it is not maintained properly, it will cease to function. It may be possible to hire the contractor on a support basis after the initial installation.

There have been reports (24) of laboratories which have abandoned LIMS development projects, such as one at a U.S. government materials testing laboratory. After working on the initial specifications for 2 years, and having no deliverable product, the contractor went out of business. The time and the money were wasted. If the contractor had been part of a team with overall responsibility for the project, it may not have failed.

Purchase a LIMS from a Vendor. All of the systems reviewed in earlier chapters should be considered candidates for purchase. It probably isn't possible to find a system which meets all of the laboratory's requirements. The decision on which system to purchase should be based on which one comes closest to meeting the requirements and which system best fits into the lab's operation. The size and complexity of the project will have an impact on which system is chosen. A PC based system will be inadequate for a medium-sized or large system. If a computer already exists on which to install the LIMS software, the selection is automatically narrowed to those vendors who support that hardware.

There have been reports (24) of laboratories which used an in-house system that evolved over several years, until finally a major rewrite was required to add the functionality of a newly purchased system. At that point, the in-house system was abandoned in favor of the purchased system. This doesn't mean that the in-house system was a failure. It means that it made sense economically to provide the additional functionality by purchasing it rather than developing it in-house. Of course, support issues may have played a large part in this decision. The LIMS vendors are in business to sell systems. This automatically implies that support and new features will be available.

A LIMS with a small scope may need only a few of the features offered by the commercial packages; thus, in-house development is an option. As we saw above, writing a medium-sized or large LIMS is a very demanding and expensive project, not to mention supporting it once implemented. Thus, the implementation of a medium-sized or large LIMS should include the purchase of a commercial LIMS package. As we describe in Chapter 15, in many cases LIMS are not ready to be used immediately after purchase. They should be considered the starting point or core system. A commercial system provides the database and the user interface, two very important aspects of the system. Tailoring and customizing the system to meet the laboratory's particular requirements must be expected. User-written code can cause the system to blend into lab operations, sometimes making the system completely transparent to the user.

The LIMS team must have members with the ability to customize the vendor's product. Help in developing this expertise can come from the vendor through training or on-site consulting. Vendor consultants can be hired for a few months to aid with installation, training, and customizing.

Computer Software System Life Span

Computer software systems have life spans and life cycles, just like machines or even living things. They are conceived, developed, born (installed), used, and they die (no longer used). Sometimes they get sick by developing bugs from ill-tested code, or by needing a new feature, and they must be cured by the doctor (modified by a programmer).

The life cycles of many computer software systems contain similar time periods during which similar activities, or functions, take place. Figure 11-3 illustrates the projected time requirements of these functions for a LIMS installation, plotted against the relative anticipated benefit.

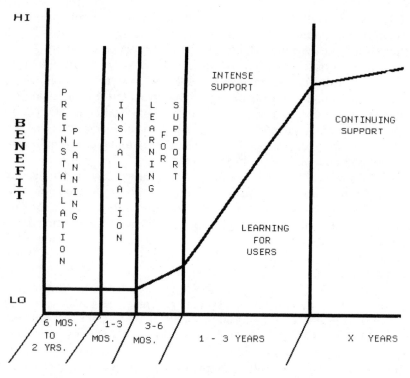

Figure 11-3. Time requirements for the LIMS life cycle.

These functions are summarized in Table 11-5. A discussion of the requirements and other considerations of each function follow.

Preinstallation Planning. Preinstallation planning has already been discussed in the above sections "Determining System Requirements and Preselection Planning" and "Selecting the LIMS Software." The latter section includes writing or contracting a system for those who choose these alternatives. The time required for preinstallation planning will vary, depending mainly on which source of software is chosen. An es-

Table 11-5. Life Cycle of a LIMS

1. Preinstallation planning (may include development)
2. Installation
3. Learning — for support personnel
4. Learning — for users
5. Intense support
6. Continued support

timated 4–6 months is needed for the initial market survey, plus additional time to finalize a purchase decision. For those writing a full-function LIMS, the first functions can be expected to be on-line and operational at the end of another 6 months. An additional year is required for the development project to near its completion.

Installation.   Installation for an in-house written LIMS will blend into the preinstallation planning function as the various LIMS functions are completed and put on-line. For a purchased system, installation will require 1-3 months. Installation for vendor systems is either included in the purchase price or is offered as an option. In most cases, allowing the vendor to install the product will decrease the time requirement.

Learning for Support Personnel.   As mentioned above, a LIMS support team will be required to implement the LIMS and provide support to all LIMS users.

The support team will begin using the system immediately following installation. Only small, selected groups of users and test methods should be set up during the first 3–6 months of use. By bringing users on-line slowly, the support team will have the time and opportunity to become familiar with the system at a controlled pace and not be faced with too much demand too soon.

Learning for Users.   The learning curve for the LIMS users is steepest during the intense support period. This is also the time during which the benefits of the project will become apparent. Thus, the faster the users learn how to use the system, the faster the benefits will be gained. Similarly, the more the users learn about the system, the more benefits will be gained. Learning by the LIMS users will be a continuing process. Users will continue to learn more about the system individually, and there will always be new users.

A commitment to provide proper LIMS training, and follow-up by the LIMS team, will pay off many times in the long run. When the system is new, many users will be breaking new ground as they use the LIMS functions to help them do their job. Sharing information about problems and solutions among users facilitates the learning process. A LIMS users group could be formed as a platform for information interchange. Anything to help or speed learning for the users is well worth the investment.

Intense Support.   As we mention later in Chapter 15, during the intense support period, four to six full-time support personnel should be available for a medium-sized or large LIMS implementation. The size and complexity of the project and the ability of the support personnel should determine the size of the team. For a very large project, six or more persons is reasonable. Project implementation should not appear to drag on forever. The users must see commitment to the system in terms of support before they will commit. Support must include training, bug fixes, instrument interfacing, addition or customization of features, and a hotline number to answer questions. Support must include having LIMS team members spend time with the users to make sure that they answer their questions and to observe the system in use. Often, simply by observing the lab members doing their jobs and using the LIMS, helpful hints can be given by the LIMS team which result in time savings.

Understaffing during the intense support period can be fatal to the project. The rate at which the LIMS is introduced into a group of laboratories must be managed. Generally, however, the faster the better. Lab analysts should not be overwhelmed with new methods, but the possibility of this happening is slim. A project management scheme should be used for bringing new methods on line, interfacing instruments, customizing data inputs and report outputs, and helping users solve specific problems.

Continued Support.   The same types of support provided during the intense support period are required during the continuing support period, only at a lower level. New users will still require training. New instruments will still require interfacing. Users will still request modifications of methods, report outputs, etc., which will require the same expertise as before.

Separating the intense and continuing support periods requires the judgment of the LIMS manager. It may occur when the number of projects on the list drops to a predefined number or when a certain set of projects are completed. Continuing support may begin when all the instruments which process large numbers of samples have been interfaced. It is not likely to begin when all the users have been trained, because, hopefully, training would be concentrated in the early intense support period.

Buy In

As described in Chapter 15, support for a LIMS should come from top management. When this happens, gaining buy-in from all lab members is much easier; however, it still requires effort. The LIMS manager will have to spend a certain amount of time obtaining buy-in from lab managers and lab analysts. The best way to obtain support from lab members is to prove that the LIMS can help them do their job. Support from top management will allow the LIMS team to install the LIMS. Support from within the lab will have to be earned. Buy-in will have to earned. It is up to the LIMS manager to determine where buy-in has and has not been obtained. In many cases, more effort will have to be applied in areas where buy-in comes slowly.

Familiarity with the LIMS, its functions, and its capabilities, and with the LIMS team and its capabilities, is prerequisite to buy-in. The LIMS users will gain familiarity with the system during training and with the LIMS team later. Lab managers should also be given the opportunity to become familiar with the LIMS. One successful method is the development of a *management overview* of the LIMS — a presentation designed to acquaint lab management with the LIMS project. After the overview is polished with a few live performances, it can be put on videotape, thus saving preparation and presentation time. The overview should contain the basics of the LIMS operation, such as the core functions of LOGIN, results entry, results verification, and results reporting. The supervisory functions of backlog, turnaround times, etc., should also be discussed, together with the reason for implementing the project. Training programs and case studies of use in particular laboratories should be described.

Buy-in will always seem to come slow. LIMS users must have a reason to buy in. Support from top management will certainly help, but the system must be able to stand alone if it is to be a success.

Summary

Many factors influence LIMS management, the most influential being the size and complexity, or scope, of the LIMS. Size is related to the number of samples processed using the LIMS in a given amount of time. Complexity is related to the number of test methods, users, and automated instruments. Determining system requirements, selecting or developing a system, and supporting the system can be managed by a team approach, with all teams led by the LIMS manager. The LIMS manager must be experienced in managing computer systems in order to manage the inevitable system changes caused by time. Resource and project management skills are also needed by the LIMS manager. And not least, the LIMS manager must also have good interpersonal skills in order to gain and sustain buy-in from management and all lab members. In short, the LIMS manager is the key to success of the project. The LIMS team must be given adequate resources and the project must be driven by top management, as we discuss further in Chapter 15.

For a laboratory embarking on a LIMS project, determining how to obtain LIMS software is perhaps the most important decision the LIMS manager and the LIMS team will have to make. And unfortunately, this decision must be made at the beginning of the project, when little is known about LIMS and when the expectations of the system are uncertain. The question of whether to write, contract, or buy a LIMS must be answered based on what is best for the particular situation and the laboratory environment. As noted, writing a LIMS is a tremendous undertaking; however, it can be done. Many labs have written their own LIMS. On the other hand, many labs with in-house LIMS are now switching to commercial packages (26).

The problems with in-house LIMS are related not to technology but to support. As stated above, support for in-house systems is often inadequate. Companies that are not in business to write, sell, and support software do not have much success in supporting large systems written in-house. Software support after installation has three requirements: (1) answering questions about the use of the software, (2) fixing bugs, and (3) providing new features. These support requirements must be met, regardless of the cost, or the system will become inadequate, out-of-date, and will surely die.

Although it is possible to write a LIMS, problems abound. These involve not only support once the system is in place, but initial implementation as well. It has been reported that up to 25% of large projects and 75% of all software projects are canceled before completion. Also, when large systems are delivered, they are, on average, 1 year late and cost twice as much as projected. Further, there is evidence that many software systems delivered are not even used (53).

With these support and delivery problems in mind, it appears that purchasing a LIMS, with subsequent customization and tailoring to blend it into the laboratory environment, is the preferred method. Commercial LIMS packages have gained the reputation of being unable to meet all the laboratory's needs. And because of the diversity of needs and situations, this reputation is true. The LIMS vendors realize that there is no way that they can meet all needs, thus, the systems of today are built to be customized, and the systems of tomorrow may even customize themselves.

Section Four

Getting the Most Out of LIMS

Chapter 12

Customization and Tailoring of LIMS

In Chapter 3 we defined the relationship between LIMS and laboratory automation by stating that LIMS functions provide a backbone on which to build laboratory automation. If we assume that this relation is fairly accurate, then it follows that installing a LIMS must not be an immediate solution to all laboratory automation needs, or nothing would have to be built. The relation implies that a LIMS still needs work after installation to achieve maximum benefit through laboratory automation.

Modifications to a LIMS which are done to make it fit better into a particular environment can be grouped into one of two categories: customization or tailoring. In Chapter 4 we noted that these two categories were similar in that they may change the appearance of the LIMS to the user and differ in the degree of change. Generally, customization is more involved, the changes are more extensive, and the execution of user-written code is usually required. Tailoring can be thought of as vendor-supplied flexibility. The amount of flexibility provided by some LIMS is extensive. Even without the use of user-written code, many functions and features can be modified virtually on-line. Some LIMS can tailor results reports, whereas others require a customized, user-written program to do so. The ability to modify the user interface screens almost completely is a tailorable feature for some LIMS but is not possible with others.

A LIMS is customized or tailored to adapt it to various changing environments. The purpose of this chapter is to illustrate customization and tailoring because of their importance to the overall concept of LIMS. Without these capabilities, laboratory automation would be much harder to achieve.

Customization

In Chapters 5,7,and 8, we looked at LIMS functionality, described as "access to user-written code," during sample LOGIN, results entry, and results reporting. Accessing user-written code from a LIMS function is the highest form of customization, as well as the most extensive. Figure 12-1 lists several tailoring and customizing techniques, including access to user-written code.

There are two primary methods of accessing user-written code. The first method involves adding a complete user-written function to the system. The function is added by inserting it into one of the LIMS menus. Once on the menu, it looks the same as any of the standard functions. Some LIMS provide a function by which menus can be edited, either to delete existing functions or to add new ones. We can generally refer to this capability as an *edit menu* function. Using this function constitutes tailoring the system. However, the functionality added to a LIMS by including user-written programs as menu items certainly constitutes customization.

	A X I O M	B EC CA KL MS A N	L I DM ES C / S M	L A HB PS A M	N ER PLL ESA OB N	2 P0 E0 0	NA EC PLC ESE OS NS	VL AI RM IS A / ND M	SM SA VMN GPA LG EE R
Tailor screen fields	X	X	X		X	X		X	X
Add totally new screens	X	X	X	X	X	X		X	X
Tailor menus	X	X	X	X	X	X	X	X	X
Tailor prompts		X	X	X	X	X	X	X	X
Tailor messages	X	X	X	X	X	X		X	X
Tailor reports	X	X	X	X	X	X	X	X	X
Add totally new reports	X	X	X	X	X	X	X	X	X
Add user-written menu items	X	X	X	X	X	X	X	X	X
Access to user-written code from LIMS functions	X	X	X	X		X	X	X	X

Figure 12-1. LIMS comparison — customization and tailoring.

Customization of LIMS/SM

The second method of customization is the access of user-written code from within one of the standard LIMS functions. The DEC LIMS/SM package offers extensive use of this functionality through three mechanisms: (1) User Event Routines, (2) User Action Routines, and (3) Data Reduction Algorithms. By using these three mechanisms and imagination, anything the LIMS does can be customized, and the LIMS can be made to do anything. The functions, forms, screens, tests, reports, menus, database retrieval, security checks, and anything else can be modified to provide any functionality the user wants.

The three mechanisms used by LIMS/SM are described below as a means of providing insight into the very important issue of LIMS customization.

User Event Routine (UER)

UERs are user-written subroutines which are associated with particular LIMS/SM functions. DEC defines UERs as "routines that can be integrated with LIMS/SM functions to adapt LIMS/SM to specific requirements of your laboratory" (54). The following is a list of LIMS/SM menus and the functions which appear on that menu to which UERs can be added:

Administrative Menu
    Enter or Edit Client Information
    Enter or Edit Project Information
    Enter or Edit Subject Information
    Enter or Edit Schedule Information

Sample Entry and Display Menu
    Log Sample
    Log Samples in Batch Mode
    Generate a New Collection List
    Receive Sample by Collection List
    Receive Sample by Individual Sample
    Generate a New Worksheet

Sample Modification Menu
    Edit Sample Information
    Add New Aliquot
    Change Aliquot Location by Sample ID
    Change Aliquot Location by Worksheet
    Change Aliquot Priority
    Cancel Test Request
    Cancel Sample

Test Results Menu
  Enter or Edit Test Results by Sample
  Enter or Edit Test Results by Test Code
  Enter or Edit Test Results by Worksheet
  Review Test Results by Sample
  Review Test Results by Test Code
  Review Test Results by Worksheet
  Approve Sample by Individual Sample
  Approve Samples for a Subject

Laboratory Setup Menu
  Enter or Edit Collector Information
  Enter or Edit Device Information
  Enter or Edit Instrument Type Information
  Enter or Edit Location Information
  Enter or Edit Route Information
  Enter or Edit ID Algorithm
  Enter or Edit Logger Information

Report Menu
  Print Sample Label

Test and Sample Setup Menu
  Enter or Edit Sample Type Information
  Enter or Edit Specific Test Information
  Enter or Edit Test Information
  Enter or Edit Test Group Information
  Enter or Edit System Mapping
  Enter or Edit Test Mapping

System Menu
  Edit Parameter Information
  Enter or Edit User Information
  Enter or Edit Menu
  Enter or Edit Function

Archive/Retrieve Menu
  Archive LIMS/SM Sample Data
  Retrieve LIMS/SM Data From Archive
  Copy LIMS/SM Data to Retrieve Database

(Functions not on a menu)
  Automatic Sample Login
  Batch Login
  Remote Add Aliquot with Results
  Remote Add Test Requests with Results

Remote Add Test Results
Remote Alter Priority
Remote Cancel Test Requests
Remote Login Sample
Remote Login Sample with Results

As we see, the number of LIMS/SM functions which can use UERs is quite extensive. Each of these functions has a specific, uniquely named UER associated with it. For example, the UER for the sample LOGIN function is UER_MLOGIN. The UER for the specific test entry or edit function is UER_SPTEST. Each UER is a function subroutine with at least one argument. Most UERs use two or three arguments for data transfer into and out of the routine. The exact structure and intended use of the subroutine arguments for each UER are described in the LIMS/SM documentation.

LIMS/SM is delivered with a default, or *dummy* UER in place for each function. The LIMS/SM user can then modify the UERs as desired. Digital makes the following statement in regard to customer customization: "You can do your own customization or contract with DIGITAL Software Services for the work. If your organization does the customization, it is fully responsible for the code and for the results the software produces" (52). This is what we should expect. No vendor can be responsible for modifications made by its customers. Digital does provide guidelines and very good documentation to aid in the customization effort. And importantly, like most other LIMS vendors, Digital offers contract customization services.

The following is a listing of the default "Enter and Edit Specific Test" function UER, UER_SPTEST (54), as delivered with the system. Note that Digital calls it a stub routine and that it "is intended for modification by the user":

```
      INTEGER*4 FUNCTION UER_SPTEST(TEST_CODE,SAMPLE_TYPE,
     1   TEST_LIMITS_TYPE, NED_FLAG, UER_MODE )
c
c+
c*******************************************************c
PURPOSE: User Event Routine (UER) for Specific Test Entry/
Edit
c
c INPUT ARGUMENTS (Read Only):
c
c TEST_CODE = The TEST_CODE of the Specific Tests Record.
c
c SAMPLE_TYPE = The SAMPLE_TYPE of the Specific Tests
```

```
c Record.
c
c TEST_LIMITS_TYPE = The TEST_LIMITS_TYPE of the Specific
c               Tests Record.
c
c (These values are only defined when UER_MODE = 1 or 2
c (see below). They are undefined at other times and
c should not be used.)
c
c NED_FLAG = Contains an ASCII character indicating what
c         operation is being performed on the record:
c
c 'N' = New record is being stored
c 'E' = Existing record being edited (data may be
c unaltered)
c 'D' = Existing record is being deleted
c
c (This value is only defined when UER_MODE = 1 or 2. It
c is undefined at other times and should not be used.)
c
c UER_MODE = Integer value passed to the UER:
c
c       1 = Before the database COMMIT
c       2 = After the database COMMIT
c       3 = Just before exiting the function
c
c FUNCTION VALUE RETURNED:
c
c When the UER_MODE = 1, this function must return an
c integer value:
c       1 = Proceed with the database COMMIT
c       2 = Cancel the COMMIT, ROLLBACK instead
c       Any other value will cause the function to abort.
c
c When the UER_MODE = 2 or 3, the function value is not
c checked, and may assume any value.
c
c
c OUTLINE:
c
c This is a stub routine supplied by Digital Equipment
c Corp., as part of the VAX LIMS/SM package, and is
c intended for modification by the user. The user is
c cautioned that any modification to the contents of the
c LIMS/SM database, LIMS/SM parameters, or LIMS/SM working
c files, within this routine will invalidate Digital's
c warranty.
```

```
C
C
C*****************************************************
C-
  CHARACTER*(*) TEST_CODE
  CHARACTER*(*) SAMPLE_TYPE
  CHARACTER*(*) TEST_LIMITS_TYPE

  CHARACTER*1 NED_FLAG
  INTEGER*4 UER_MODE

  UER_SPTEST = 1          ! proceed with the COMMIT
  RETURN
  END
```

Although some UERs are called only once or twice, a UER is usually called at three different points during processing of the associated LIMS/SM function. These points are:

1. Pre-COMMIT. The UER is called after all the information is filled in on the screen but before committing it to the database.
2. Post-COMMIT. The UER is called after the information filled in by the user has been committed to the database.
3. Function Exit. The UER is called just before the LIMS function exits.

In the above UER program listing, the variable UER_MODE is set by LIMS/SM to either 1, 2, or 3 and is passed to the UER to indicate from which point the UER is being called. When running at the pre-COMMIT point, UER_MODE = 1, when running at the post-COMMIT point, UER_MODE = 2, and when running at the function exit point, UER_MODE = 3. The UER can perform different functions at the different points, or it can merely return without doing anything at certain points, depending on what it needs to do. Figure 12-2 presents a flowchart of LIMS/SM function processing. This flowchart illustrates the three call points as locations in the flow.

An actual customized UER is presented in Appendix C-1.

User Action Routine (UAR)

The LIMS/SM system user interface is built on Digital's Forms Management System (FMS). FMS, which is a Digital *layered product,* provides a user interface to an application by the use of full-screen forms. LIMS/SM uses one or more FMS forms with each LIMS function. An

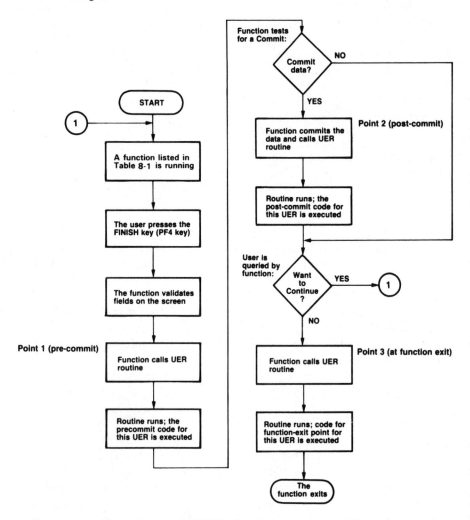

Figure 12-2. Flowchart of LIMS/SM function processing. (Digital Equipment Corp. 1987. *VAX LIMS/SM Manager's Guide.* Maynard, Mass. p. 9-3)

FMS form can have any number of fields defined and displayed for the terminal user to fill in. Each form has several user definable parameters associated with it. The form parameters include form name, colors, width, ruler, and user action routines. The UARs are user-written sub-routines which are called at different times while the form is being displayed. One particular UAR is associated with programming the terminal function keys and is called just before the form is initially displayed.

Other UARs are called in conjunction with using the help features of FMS.

Each field of a form has several user-definable parameters associated with it. These field parameters include field name, help text, integrity checks such as numeric or alphabetic, default value, display only, reverse video, and user action routines. The UARs are user-written function subroutines which are called whenever the user completes data input to the field. LIMS/SM allows the addition of UARs to any of the FMS forms and to any field of any form. Each field can have up to 15 UARs defined.

An actual UAR is presented in Appendix C-2.

Data Reduction Algorithm (DRA)

DRAs are user-written function subroutines which are called each time a LIMS/SM user enters or changes a test result. DRAs are defined to LIMS/SM in conjunction with the "Specific Test Entry/Edit (STEE)" function. In LIMS/SM the concept of *specific test* is a combination of three components: (1) test code, (2) sample type, and (3) test limits type. The specific test is necessary because any physical or analytical test may be run on many different sample types and may require a different set of limits for each sample type. Thus, any one test code may be associated with an unlimited number of specific tests, and each specific test can have a different DRA defined. Figure 12-3 shows the LIMS/SM STEE screen form. On it, the first four fields are test code, sample type, test limits type, and reduction algorithm. The reduction algorithm field is where the name of the DRA function subroutine is entered. The particular specific test illustrated is for the "ASH" test, "MISC" sample type, and "NORMAL" test limits. The DRA for this specific test is "DRA_ASH."

DRAs, defined using the STEE function, are actually used in conjunction with the three LIMS/SM "Enter or Edit Test Results (EETR)" functions. These three functions are "EETR-by Sample," "EETR-by Test Code," and "EETR-by Worksheet." The EETR functions call the appropriate DRA whenever a test result is entered or changed. Typically, DRAs are used to calculate a final result from intermediate results, raw data, or test component values. In other words, an analyst entering test results would enter some of the raw data, and then the final result(s) would be calculated by the DRA. Figure 12-4 illustrates the "EETR-by Sample" function being used to enter test results for the "ASH" test for sample "P-ASH-RM10." In this example, the analyst entering the results keyed in the first four numbers, which are "25.0," "30.0,"

148 Getting the Most Out of LIMS

```
         Test Code:            ASH
         Sample Type:          MISC
         Test Limits Type:     NORMAL
         Reduction Algorithm:  DRA_ASH


         Required Sample Size:        100
         Required Size Units:  GRAMS
```

Press <PF2> once for HELP on the current field, twice for HELP on the screen

Figure 12-3. DEC LIMS/SM specific test entry/edit screen for the ASH/MISC/NORMAL Specific Test.

Sample ID: **P-ASH-RM10**

Aliquot ID	Test Code	Run Number	Component Code	Result Flag	Text Flag	Result
P	ASH	1	TARE_WGT			25.0
P	ASH	1	GROSS_WGT			30.0
P	ASH	1	FINAL_WGT			27.0
P	ASH	1	NO_CYCLES			2
P	ASH	1	TEMP			600
P	ASH	1	CRUC_TYPE			PORCELAIN
P	ASH	1	ASH_TYPE			OXIDE
P	ASH	1	%ASH			40.00

Reason for change:

Press <PF2> once for HELP on the current field, twice for HELP on the screen

Figure 12-4. DEC LIMS/SM test result entry — by sample screen for sample "P-ASH-RM10".

"27.0," and "2." The DRA then filled in "600," "porcelain," and "oxide," as default values and calculated the final result of "40.00"%.
The actual "DRA_ASH" subroutine is presented in Appendix C-3.

Tailoring

As indicated above, tailoring a LIMS can be considered a form of vendor-supplied flexibility. Tailoring is generally not as involved or complicated as customizing, but it can still have a great impact on making a LIMS fit into a particular environment. Much of what we might consider tailoring could also be thought of as LIMS setup, which was discussed in Chapter 9. Tailoring usually involves on-line modifications to menus, prompts, queries, prompt language, screen forms, and report formats.

A major feature provided by most LIMS is the ability to tailor the individual menus for each user. This capability, discussed in Chapter 9, provides for a streamlined operation as well as for security. If a user doesn't need to use a particular LIMS function for whatever reason, then there is no reason for that function to appear on her or his menu list.

The PE-Nelson LIMS 2000 and ACCESS*LIMS products possess extensive report generation flexibility, although they provide it quite differently. LIMS 2000 allows an ad hoc database query command sequence to be saved for repeated use. ACCESS*LIMS provides the capability through purchase of an option from the Oracle database supplier.

Tailoring LIMS/SM

To illustrate LIMS tailoring, we will again use DEC's LIMS/SM for examples. Like most LIMS, LIMS/SM provides the capability to tailor screens, queries (or prompts), messages, and menus, as described below.

Screens. Both data entry and help screens can be readily modified in LIMS/SM. As stated above, LIMS/SM uses DEC's FMS to provide screen forms. (FMS uses the term *form* and LIMS/SM uses the term *screen.* It is sometimes appropriate to use them together as *screen form,* but all three are probably interchangeable.) Any screen can be modified using the FMS screen editor. There are certain required fields that cannot be removed. A screen (or form) is copied from the forms library, edited, and copied back to the library, replacing the old copy.

Queries. Queries are those questions or prompts that appear on data-entry screens when LIMS/SM needs to get further information from the user about how to proceed. Examples of queries are 'Client not found, want to add a new one? [Y/N]' and 'Do you want to repeat? [Y/N]' (54). Queries need to be tailored in order to change default responses or when certain LIMS/SM terms have been changed, such as using the word *customer* instead of *client*. In the case of such a term substitution, the appropriate data entry and help screens would also have to be modified.

LIMS/SM uses approximately 60 queries. Table 12-1 lists some of them. The queries are maintained as records in the LIMS/SM database. They are modified using DBQ, the VAX DBMS query language. An example of a DBQ session is presented below. The purpose of this session is to change the term *technician* to *analyst,* and to change the default response from "N" to "Y."

```
$DBQ
dbq> BIND LIMSSM$DATABASE:LIMSSMSC
dbq> READY SERVICE_AREA EXCLUSIVE UPDATE
dbq> FETCH FIRST QUERIES USING QUE_QUERY_ID
QUE_QUERY_ID [X(16)]=LIMSSM$_Q_MST123
QUE_QUERY_ID = LIMSSM$_Q_MST123
QUE_CHANGE_DATE = 12-OCT-1984 16:31:12:32
QUE_CHANGE_OPERATOR = 999999
QUE_QUERY_TEXT = Do you want to add a new technician? [Y/
N]
QUE_QUERY_REPLYS(1) = Y
QUE_QUERY_REPLYS(2) = N
QUE_QUERY_REPLYS(3) =
QUE_QUERY_REPLYS(4) =
QUE_QUERY_REPLYS(5) =
QUE_DEFAULT = 2
QUE_DEFAULT_TIMEOUT = 2
dbq> MODIFY QUE_QUERY_TEXT
QUE_QUERY_TEXT[X(69)] = Do you want to add a new analyst?
             [Y/N]
dbq> MODIFY QUE_DEFAULT
QUE_DEFAULT [FIXED] = 1
dbq> COMMIT
dbq> EXIT
$
```

Messages. LIMS/SM uses approximately 800 messages to communicate actions, errors, and many other kinds of information the user. The messages are kept in a text file, which can be edited using any VAX editor. Any message can be changed. After the change is made, the message file is compiled using the VAX/VMS System Message Utility,

Table 12-1. LIMS/SM Queries
     (Digital Equipment Corporation. 1987. *VAX LIMS/SM Planning Workbook*. Maynard, Mass.)

Query ID	Query Text and Default Responses
LIMSSM$_Q_ARC003	Autobackup is ON. Do you want to continue? [Y/N] - Default: 1 Default if Timeout: 2
LIMSSM$_Q_ASU001	Do you want to see Completed, Reviewed, or Both? [C/R/B] - Default: 3 Default if Timeout: 3
LIMSSM$_Q_CAS001	Do you really want to cancel this sample? [Y/N] - Default: 2 Default if Timeout: 2
LIMSSM$_Q_CAT001	Do you want to cancel selected Test Requests? [Y/N] - Default: 1 Default if Timeout: 2
LIMSSM$_Q_CLI001	Client not found, want to add a new one? [Y/N] - Default: 1 Default if Timeout: 2
LIMSSM$_Q_CLL001	Collection List generated. Press <RETURN> to continue. Default: 0 Default if Timeout: 0
LIMSSM$_Q_COL001	Collector not found, want to add a new one? [Y/N] - Default: 1 Default if Timeout: 2
LIMSSM$_Q_DEV001	Device not found, want to add a new one? [Y/N] - Default: 1 Default if Timeout: 2
LIMSSM$_Q_DIR001	Do you want to cancel? [Y/N] - Default: 1 Default if Timeout: 1
LIMSSM$_Q_DIR002	Do you want to save a copy of this directory? [Y/N] - Default: 2 Default if Timeout: 2
LIMSSM$_Q_DIR003	Screen output limit reached. Do you want to go to the top? [Y/N] - Default: 1 Default if Timeout: 1
LIMSSM$_Q_GEN001	Do you want to continue? [Y/N] - Default: 1 Default if Timeout: 2
LIMSSM$_Q_GEN002	Do you want to Repeat, Continue, or Exit? [R/C/E] - Default: 1 Default if Timeout: 3

Table 12-2. LIMS/SM Messages (file listing)

```
_GEN014  <DEVICE does not exist>.
_GEN015  <INSTRUMENT TYPE does not exist>
_GEN016  <COLLECTOR does not exist>
_GEN017  <SAMPLE TYPE does not exist>
_GEN018  <Invalid numeric>
_GEN019  <ALGORITHM does not exist>
_GEN020  <SYSTEM does not exist>
_GEN021  <KEY fields cannot be edited>
_GEN022  <CLIENT/PROJECT combination does not exist>
_GEN023  <COMPONENT CODE does not exist>
_GEN024  <COLLECTION LIST does not exist>
_GEN025  <WORKSHEET does not exist>
_GEN026  <Past end of data list, input not allowed>
_GEN027  <ROUTE does not exist>
_GEN028  <Invalid Action Code: enter A, D, U or R>
_GEN029  <Test Request has been changed by another user>
_GEN030  <No Test Requests with results to review>
_GEN031  <Beyond end of list, cannot go to next page>
_GEN032  <STOP DATE precedes START DATE>
_GEN033  <Test Request not complete yet; cannot change Code>
_GEN034  <Report Destination Type must be Print, File or Mail (P, F or M)>
_GEN035  <Client !AS is not currently active>/FAO_COUNT=1
_GEN036  <Test Request not available for review>
_GEN037  <Test Code must be an individual test, not a group>
_GEN038  <An ID or Name cannot be entered in addition to ALL>
_GEN039  <CLIENT ID required to continue>
_GEN040  <COMPONENT CODE required to continue>
_GEN041  <Cannot delete; linked to Schedule or Subjects>
_GEN042  <Cannot edit Subject ID>
_GEN043  <DEVICE ID required to continue>
_GEN044  <END DATE must be after START DATE>
_GEN045  <Flag required to continue>
_GEN046  <INSTRUMENT TYPE required to continue>
_GEN047  <Invalid response; enter Y. or N>
```

and then *linked* into the LIMS/SM message handler. Table 12-2 lists a portion of the message file. A reason to modify a message might be to change terminology, such as changing all occurrences of *client* to *customer*.

Menus. LIMS/SM consists of some 20 menus. From these menus the approximately 60 system functions, and any user added functions, are selected for execution. Figure 12-5 illustrates the default LIMS/SM menu *tree structure*. The structure can be rearranged by the user by modifying which functions and submenus appear on which menu. In addition, new menus can be created by the user. Menus are modified or added using the "Enter or Edit Menu Function".

Tailoring ACCESS*LIMS

ACCESS*LIMS uses Oracle's database product. Just as the query database definition was changed above for LIMS/SM, similar changes can be made to the ACCESS*LIMS database definitions using SQL*Plus,

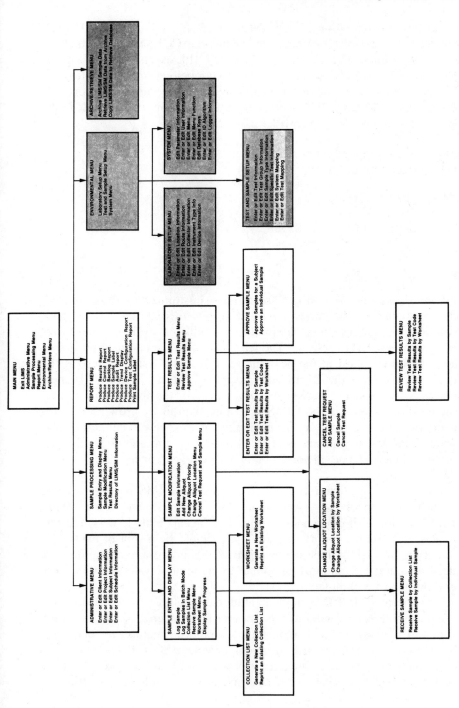

Figure 12-5. Default LIMS/SM menu tree structure (Digital Equipment Corp. 1987. *VAX LIMS/SM Planning Workbook.* Maynard, Mass. p. 5-3)

Oracle's implementation of SQL (Structured Query Language). The following SQL session illustrates modifying an ACCESS*LIMS database using SQL*Plus. The caption SAMPLE_TYPE is changed to PRODUCT_FORMULATION for everyone who belongs to the datagroup PLASTICS. As a result of the modification, all queries and reports for the datagroup PLASTICS will contain the caption PRODUCT_FORMULATION instead of SAMPLE_TYPE.

```
CREATE VIEW PLASTICS
(PRODUCT_FORMULATION)
AS
SELECT SAMPLE_TYPE
FROM SAMPLE
WHERE DATAGROUP = 'PLASTICS'
```

Summary

Future generations of LIMS will require less customization to accomplish the modifications that now require it. Links to external software, instrument interfacing, report flexibility, etc., will become easier and better with each new LIMS release. The features which the end user must now add will be standard in the near future. But this doesn't mean that the need to customize the LIMS will disappear. There will always be new horizons to view and new goals to achieve. In the foreseeable future, the need to customize the LIMS will more than likely grow rather than decrease. We are now at the beginning of this new technology trek, which includes the management of all information in and about the laboratory. Features and customizations not yet even conceived will someday be standard.

Enhancing the tailorability of the commercial LIMS products should be near the top of the "opportunities for improvement" list of every LIMS vendor. Tailoring should be simple. The capability to design forms, menus, data paths, report formats, etc., should be a tool of every lab. Tailoring the system must become part of the day-to-day operation. The need for computer support personnel to maintain day-to-day LIMS operation must be eliminated.

As experience in LIMS implementation and usage grows, LIMS users are becoming accustomed to the fact that some degree of customization is required. As a result, customization and tailoring features are becoming very important in distinguishing among LIMS. LIMS users and potential users have begun comparing packages based on these features. Systems that do not offer relatively easy customization will not succeed. Building flexibility into the LIMS is not a trivial undertaking. Use of existing and emerging standards in communications, database technology, windowing, etc., should make the task easier. Each system will, of course, contain different mechanisms of implementation. Those systems which offer the best and easiest modification schemes will, without exception, gain a larger customer base than those which do not.

Chapter 13

LIMS Training — Getting the Most for Your Money

Computer Training — General Considerations

Good people deserve good training, and good systems deserve good training (51).

Investing in a software system without training is like building a swimming pool when you and/or your children don't know how to swim. You can still use either, but not to its fullest. Training is needed for two reasons:

1. To make sure that users get the most from the investment.
2. To reduce the support requirement.

In the case of the pool, you can't get full enjoyment from its use if you can't go into the deep end. In the case of computer software, you can't get the full benefit of its use if you don't know how to use all its features. If your children know how to swim, the requirement for direct supervision when they play near the pool will be much less than if they cannot swim. The more software users know about its use, the less support they require.

Employers have always helped their employees learn new skills by utilizing various methods of training. As computers and computer software have become common in business, so has computer training. In the 1960s, computer training consisted of either operations training or learning programming languages, such as FORTRAN, BASIC, or assembly language. In the early 1970s, training focused on more programming languages, new languages, more assembly language, and new programming techniques. By the mid-1970s, users began to expect and plan for training of in-house written and purchased application software. By 1980, computer training included on-line computer assisted methods. And now, as a part of any new software addition, the consideration of training comes naturally. Vendor and third-party training is offered both on-site and off-site. Consultants who teach others the methods of computer training are available. Company training departments have geared up for computer training in the past few years and now employ computer training professionals.

The question today is not "Do we do computer training?" but rather "What is the best method of computer training and how much is required?" The answer to today's question is, unfortunately, "It all depends." It depends on previous familiarity with computer methods, how much needs to be learned, how much time is required to learn it, and how much time is available. (Note that the whole answer did not include the phases "computer literate" or "computer illiterate," which we are all probably tired of hearing.)

LIMS Training

LIMS training can be divided into two general categories: LIMS manager training (or advanced user training) and general end-user training. We will first assume that the LIMS manager, and all the LIMS team members, are fully trained and ready to install the system. LIMS manager training will be considered in a later section.

Any training system will evolve to include new features as they are added and to smooth the presentation from class to class. There is probably no single best way to accomplish LIMS training. It requires a combination of classwork, hands-on exercises, and continuing one-on-one help after the classes are over. The following sections present some hints on how to conduct LIMS training. The suggestions presented here come from watching a successful LIMS training program which now has several hundred graduates.

There Is a Difference

Training LIMS users differs in one particular way from most other forms of computer software training. Many of the individuals who will be using LIMS will already have experience with PCs, home computers, departmental minis, or laboratory computers; however, many will have no experience. It can be assumed that most young laboratory scientists will have computer experience, as well as a large fraction of older scientists and lab technicians. But this still leaves a considerable fraction of potential LIMS users, scientists, technicians, and plant operators, with no computer experience. Thus, the LIMS training in which they will be expected to participate will likely be their first hands-on experience with a keyboard. This circumstance presents no significant problems that cannot be overcome. In fact, many of these inexperienced individuals will probably delight in the opportunity to participate in computer training. It might even open the door for future computer training.

Customized Modules and Organized Classes

Every laboratory and every LIMS installation is different. Some users will be sample submitters and log samples into the LIMS; others will enter test results as part of testing lab duties. Other users will log samples and enter test results. Some laboratories will use barcodes, automated instrumentation, and many other unique processes which others outside the lab will have no need to learn. Consequently, different users of the same system will need to know different things related to LIMS use.

A LIMS training program consisting of customized modules is recommended. Training classes and training modules should be organized by a combination of factors such as computer experience, laboratory requirements, types of instrumentation, and the test methods which will be used by the trainees once they are back on the job. For example, including one individual with no computer experience in a class of persons with a great deal of experience is not desirable. If this individual is given the extra attention required, the progress of the whole class will be impeded. If this individual is not given extra attention, she or he will suffer and probably not learn anything about using LIMS. Persons with the same level of experience must be grouped together. Another useful practice is to include members of one laboratory in a training class and teach them using the same test methods and procedures that they will be using on the job. These are examples of class organization which must be considered when scheduling training.

An example of a customized training module is one that teaches the use of barcode labels with the LIMS. Anyone not dealing with barcode labels would not need the module. Another example would be to teach the use of a particular data acquisition system, and how it interacts with the LIMS, only to those using that system. Individual modules should be based on unique applications and lab procedures.

Hands-On Training

Anytime computer training is being taught, the preferred method, whenever possible, is hands-on. For a LIMS, training should be done step by step, giving the trainees ample time between steps to try to perform what is being taught. Sample LOGIN, for example, should be demonstrated by the instructor on a terminal and then practiced by the class.

As we mention below, there are other times when other methods of teaching LIMS concepts are desired. Generally, however, each LIMS function, feature, twist, and turn should be taught by demonstrations followed by individual practice.

Ideally, one student per terminal is best, and no more than two should ever be allowed. Hands-on training when two are sharing a single terminal can be successful if the exercises are designed to allow users to take turns at the keyboard. Trying to share terminals in a class which is designed for a 1-to-1 student/terminal ratio can be a disaster. What will happen is that students with no computer experience will try to encourage their partners to do all the work, especially if the partners are somewhat familiar with a keyboard. Even when an exercise is designed for two at a terminal, this can still be a problem and must be carefully and tactfully prevented by the instructor.

Off-the-Job Navigational Training

LIMS training should be done off the job in a comfortable training room-type setting. Even with a good instructor's best efforts to make the students feel comfortable, some will be very intimidated by the new system. Some will be afraid of a keyboard. Serve them coffee and donuts, tell some jokes, and show them that they can't "break" the computer. Whatever can be done to make the students more comfortable should be done. The main thing to tell them from the beginning is that the purpose of the LIMS, and the LIMS team, is to provide them with a tool to do their jobs better. Some of them won't believe it at first, and some may never believe it, but because it's true, this should be stated several times.

There are several ways in which LIMS training can be done. One way is training on the job at the work site. This, however, has been ruled out. Another way is to train the lab supervisors and have them, in turn, train others who will be using the system. Still another way is to train selected lab analysts from each group and let them train the others. But in either case, the results would be the same. People tend to learn subjectively. Each person would learn only a few features of the LIMS, whatever looked interesting. Then, when showing what they learned to others, the same filtering would occur. This is like building a bookshelf by carefully measuring the first shelf and then using it to measure the second, the second to measure the third, and so on. By the time the last shelf is cut, it probably will not even be close in size to the first shelf.

Everyone who is expected to use the LIMS should receive training. Even lab managers who might never use it should be trained so that they can understand what their staff members are required to do. The instruction should be navigational by design. Teach how to navigate the system; don't use cookbook methods. Teach how the system works and why. The trainer must strive to make sure that there are as few misunderstandings as possible. Inevitably, some will occur, and the LIMS team will need to work closely with every individual regularly, on the job, after the training is done to help resolve problems.

Planning the Training

The first step in instituting a training program is to consider who should plan the training. The LIMS manager should play the major role in making this decision. As we will see in Chapter 11, the LIMS manager must play a leading role in most areas, and overall LIMS implementation should be done by a team, with the LIMS manager as the team leader. The LIMS manager is ultimately responsible for training preparation, but, he or she may choose to delegate responsibility to other team members. In some organizations, a training department may be available to help with training considerations and preparations. Regardless of who is doing the planning, a team approach should be used. LIMS team members and training department members are natural candidates for this team. If a commercial LIMS is being used, the vendor's representative should also be included in the initial planning as a support member of the team. As shown in Figure 13-1, LIMS vendors consider training an important aspect of their product's success. In addition, some vendors offer on-site, customized training. By all means, include anyone in the planning process who has previous experience in customizing LIMS training.

Training Time Requirements

The customized module approach aids in determining how much time will be required for training. The time needed for each module can be calculated fairly accurately, and the total time required will be the sum of the individual modules. Of course, any module taught to a group that has relatively little computer experience will naturally take longer than when taught to more experienced users. The first segment of any program being taught to a group unfamiliar with the computer system will need to cover basics such as how to log on to the computer, how to change passwords, and even how to use the keyboard. These factors must be factored into the time requirement calculation. An optimum time requirement for the training must be found. A serious flaw in much of industry training is that trainees perceive classes as too lengthy. The

LIMS training class for general users should be no more than one day long. Of course, two days are better than three, and a half day is better than a whole day, assuming that the same amount of information is taught and learned.

As older modules are revised and new ones are created, follow-up training can be offered to selected individuals or groups in need of the particular training. For example, a new training module may be developed to cover the new LIMS features included in a revision. The trainees would be existing LIMS users, and the time requirement would be substantially less. This type of follow-up training could be done as a lecture rather than as hands-on training, thus allowing more users to attend the presentation and reducing the number of times it must be given.

Once computer training for a particular software application has begun, it needs to be completed as quickly as possible. This is probably true for training of any type. A long period of training makes it hard for the student to maintain the concentration and interest necessary to obtain the maximum benefit. For example, 10 hours of training is much more effective if done in two 5-hour sessions on consecutive days compared to five 2-hour sessions.

When Should Training Be Done?

LIMS training should be done at approximately the same time that the individual would be expected to begin using the system. It should never be done too soon. It is better to have the LIMS and the particular methods

	A X I O M	B EC CA KL MS A N	L I DM ES C / S M	L A HB PS A M	N ER PLL ESA OB N	2 P0 E0 0	NA EC PLC ESE OS NS	VL AI RM IS A / ND M	SM SA VMN GPA LG EE R
Vendor training for LIMS managers	X	X	X	X		X	X	X	X
Vendor training for LIMS users	X	X	X	X	X	X	X	X	X
Vendor training off-site	X	X	X	X	X	X	X	X	X
Vendor training on-site & customized	X	X	X	X		X	X	X	X

Figure 13-1. LIMS comparison — training related.

that the individual will employ, in place and ready to use before scheduling the training. Training before the system is ready can result in the need for retraining.

How Should Outside Training Be Used?

As noted in Figure 13-1, significant training is available from the LIMS vendors. With a commercial LIMS, outside training should be used whenever possible. If there is an exact match between the vendor's system and the needs of the laboratory, vendor training is a possibility. A vendor representative should definitely be consulted by the LIMS team to find out what training is available and how the vendor can help in meeting training requirements. Vendor-customized training is an option which should be examined carefully.

There are several problems with depending totally on vendor training. The first is obviously the cost. When vendor training is used, in-house course development costs are eliminated. The costs associated with training are related either to travel to the vendor's location or to bringing in a vendor trainer to teach on-site. Bringing the vendor in is less expensive than sending a whole class to the vendor's location, but in order for the training to be cost effective, a fairly large number of people must participate. It is difficult to provide a 1-to-1 or even 2-to-1 student/terminal ratio in large classes. Also, when considering using the vendor to teach a customized on-site course, one must consider how the course will be maintained and updated when needed. It is very likely that each class will need to be different. Depending on a vendor to know how to make the necessary course modifications is probably asking too much.

Training at the vendor's location will not be customized to the students' particular needs; a LIMS team member should therefore take the vendor's off-site training to evaluate the program and to get ideas about presentation and content which might be used in building an in-house course. Participating in the vendor's training will also help uncover any misunderstandings which might exist in the use of particular LIMS functions. Sampling the vendor's training may prove to be the best use of the vendor's offerings.

Who Is the Best Instructor for LIMS Training?

Ideally, LIMS training should be done by a member of the LIMS team. If the training department is used, the course will probably become outdated. As we have said, the classes will be different because of different training modules, different laboratory needs, and other reasons. The LIMS team is in the best position to see the changes which have taken place. The trainer should take advantage of each class to learn what problems the users have with the LIMS and to take these problems back to the team for solutions.

The instructor must know how to use the LIMS expertly. It is important to create enthusiasm in the class, maintain it, and motivate the students to learn. These qualifications may be hard to find in a LIMS team member. Certainly, each member will know the LIMS sufficiently, but that doesn't imply the ability to teach it. Good teachers are a special breed. On the other hand, the possibility of training someone from the training department in LIMS and keeping that person familiar with the system is unlikely. It is better to train the LIMS team members to understand teaching techniques than to train a teacher to understand the LIMS.

The training classes should be designed to be taught by one instructor. However, the most efficient training classes will use two instructors, one to present the new material and one to circulate and help the students solve the mechanical problems associated with entering the right commands at the right time. This two-instructor approach is almost a requirement when the class consists of first-time computer users. There should always be at least two members of the LIMS team capable of conducting the training classes. Because of illness, and for many other reasons, the team must always have backup training support.

Pilot Training Classes

At the beginning, dress rehearsals of the training course should take the form of pilot training classes. At least two pilot classes should be scheduled with a small number of students per class (three or four). The students should be told at the beginning that they are "guinea pigs" for the training development, and they should probably be rescheduled for another class. Pilot training will take the pressure off the instructors to perform correctly the first time and will benefit the program in the end. The problems can be eliminated from the training program in a systematic manner before the actual training begins.

LIMS Manager Training

The preceding sections have dealt with training for general LIMS users. Their training requirement is different from that of the LIMS team. The LIMS manager and all the members of the LIMS team must know the complete details of setting up and managing, tailoring, and customizing the system — details which the general users don't need to know. Some vendors separate this type of user from others as an advanced user and offer both LIMS manager and advanced user training. But regardless of what it is called, the LIMS team should take whatever training is offered. Most of this training will occur at the vendor's location, but some of it may also be done by the vendor on-site during system installation.

Summary

Most industries now view computer training as necessary, and there should be no problem in obtaining support for LIMS training. This training may be the first computer-related training for many potential LIMS users. It should be considered an opportunity for these first-time users to become familiar with using a computer and might encourage them to learn other computer applications.

LIMS training is best accomplished by in-house teaching using customized training modules. Members of the LIMS team are in the best position to provide and maintain the training. These and the other ideas and suggestions discussed in this chapter have one common goal: to provide training in a way that will minimize the LIMS investment. Investing in LIMS means investing in a new technology of which LIMS is a part. LIMS training is not an end in itself. As the new technology develops, there will be additional opportunities for training.

Chapter 14

Validation of Computer Systems

The first section of this chapter provides a chronological description of a sampling of work and publications which document milestones along the path out of confusion in the 1970s to the current understanding of validation concepts. This section also provides a general overview of the purpose of computer system validation and of which computer systems require validation. The next section presents a working definition of computer systems validation by examining the work of R.C. Branning. A subsequent section describes the *validation life cycle* approach to computer systems validation.

The components of a computer system which can cause failure or unexpected behavior, and which represent the real reasons for computer system validation, are discussed in this chapter. Other sections examine validation concepts in conjunction with LIMS and how LIMS might be validated.

Background and General Overview

The need to validate computer related applications was documented in 1976 in Section 211.68 of the "Current GMPs in the Manufacture, processing, Packing, or Molding of Large-Volume Parenterals" (11) (listed in Figure 14-1), as pointed out by Chapman, Harris, Bluhm, and Errico (12). These authors also state that even after the 1976 Current GMP, "no one could clearly define exactly what such validation would entail," indicating that there was confusion within the industries touched by regulation. There was also uncertainty in defining which systems required validation and in understanding exactly what industry's responsibilities were.

In 1983, the Food and Drug Administration (FDA) published the *Guide to Inspection of Computerized Systems in Drug Processing* (10), referred to as the *Bluebook*. This publication's stated purpose is "to provide the field investigator with a framework upon which to build an inspection

(a) Automatic, mechanical, or electronic equipment
or other types of equipment, including computers,
or related systems that will perform a function
satisfactorily, may be used in the manufacture,
processing, packing, and holding of a drug product.
If such equipment is so used, it shall be routinely
calibrated, inspected, or checked according to a
written program designed to assure proper
performance. Written records of those calibration
checks and inspections shall be maintained.
(b) Appropriate controls shall be exercised over
computer or related systems to assure that changes
in master production and control records or other
records are instituted only by authorized
personnel. Input to and output from the computer
or related system of formulas or other records or
data shall be checked for accuracy. A backup file
of data entered into the computer or related system
shall be maintained except where certain data, such
as calculations performed in connection with
laboratory analysis, are eliminated by
computerization or other automated processes. In
such instances a written record of the program
shall be maintained along with appropriate
validation data. Hard copy or alternative systems,
such as duplicates, tapes, or microfilm, designed
to assure that backup data are exact and complete
and that it is secure from alteration, inadvertent
erasures, or loss shall be maintained.

Figure 14-1. Section 211.68 of CGMP for drug production manufacturing.

of drug establishments which utilize computer systems." The *Bluebook* and other publications by the FDA and FDA employees (13-16) seem to be particularly concerned with computer systems that are directly involved with drug manufacturing, such as process control computer systems. Process control related phrases and descriptions such as *computerized process control, computers to control drug production, drug production under computer surveillance or control, input/output devices, signal converters, distributed control, process control programs* and *process variables* are prevalent in these writings. Thus, the importance of computer systems controlling drug manufacturing processes had become obvious to the FDA by the early 1980s, and rightly so.

In 1984, the Pharmaceutical Manufacturers Association (PMA) created a subcommittee to develop a written advisory on the subject of validation. After 2 years of work, in May 1986, the PMA's Computer System Validation Committee (CSVC) published its paper, "Validation Concepts for Computer Systems Used in the Manufacture of Drug Products" (17). This paper extended the definition of which computer systems should be validated by stating, "When computers are used to process data related to the manufacture or the quality assurance of a product, it is appropriate to validate the computer systems involved.''

In 1987, the FDA published the *Technical Reference on Software Development Activities,* the second reference "designed to assist the investigator in his/her understanding of computerized systems and their controls" (18). In this publication the FDA plainly states its view concerning computer systems as follows: "The use of computerized systems to perform process control and quality assurance activities within the industries regulated by the Food and Drug Administration is becoming more prevalent as the size and cost of this technology decreases.... As these systems become instrumental in assuring the quality, safety, and integrity of FDA regulated products, it becomes extremely important for the Agency to verify that proper controls were employed to assure the correct performance and monitoring of the system once it has been installed." In this statement, as in the PMA's paper, we again see references not only to process control systems but to others as well.

Figure 14-2 lists the important publications in regard to computer system validation, chronologically ordered, and indicates their significance, as described above.

Experienced systems analysts would agree that every computer system, regardless of its function, and including both the hardware and software components, must be validated. Norbert Kuzel states, "The basic purpose of validation is to produce sufficient evidence that a computer system does what it purports to do in a reliable manner, has done so in the past, and will continue to do so in the future" (19). This account is very similar to the PMA CSVC's purpose for validation (17). (Kuzel was a member of the CSVC.) He also suggests that the operation of some computers is less "critical" than that of others and thus does not

```
    1. FDA, 1976, "CGMPs for Drug Production Manufacturing"(11);
        pointed out the need to validate computer related
applications.

    2. FDA, 1983, "Guide to Inspection of Computerized Systems
in Drug Processing"(10); primarily describes those
computer sytems used for pharmaceutical manufacturing
process control.

    3. PMA, 1986, "Validation Concepts for Computer Systems Used
        in the Manufacture of Drug Products"(17); extended
definition of "validatable" computer systems to include
those used for quality assurance.

    4. FDA, 1987, "Technical Reference on Software Development
Activities"(18); references to computer systems other      than
those used for manufacturng process control.
```

Figure 14-2. Computer systems validation — significant publications.

require the same extent of validation (19). Generally, the amount of attention given to the validation of a computer system is proportional to the degree of consequence should the system make an error.

What Is Computer System Validation?

What Is It?

Validation is not something done during an FDA (or other regulatory agency) inspection. It is not the responsibility of the regulatory agency. It is the responsibility of the food and drug product manufacturing industry. Of course, the ultimate purpose of validation of computer systems is to ensure that computers function reliably in the production of high-quality drug- and food-related products. "Validation is only one of a number of quality assurance measures" used to protect the fitness-for-use of a product (19). We have stated that the reason to validate a computer system is to "produce sufficient evidence" that the system does what it is supposed to do. It then follows that validation itself is the process of producing such evidence.

The evidence takes the form of documentation. A.S. Clark states that "documentation should not be undertaken with the sole purpose of showing an FDA investigator that the system is well designed and properly validated. Instead, the primary purpose of documentation is to facilitate communication among those who must run the system, those who must maintain the system, and those who must implement changes in the system" (14).

R.C. Branning (55) describes the validation concept as consisting of the following two components:

1. A standard operating procedure (SOP) for computer systems validation — the "what to do"
2. A validation protocol — the "how to do it"

The following descriptions of the SOP and the validation protocol are, for the most part, quotations from the cited work of Branning (55). To date, there is no magic formula that guarantees regulation compliance. The concepts described here suggest a minimum number of activities/ documentation. Actual situations and circumstances will dictate which aspects of these concepts should be given the most attention. Branning's ideas are stated briefly and to the point. They illustrate that the task of computer system validation doesn't require a magic formula, just a lot of work.

The SOP

Objective. "A limited objective could be to validate only those computer systems directly related to the production of pharmaceuticals; the broadest one would be to validate all computer systems regardless of their application. Usually it is somewhere between the two. The scope will be determined by the company philosophy, organizational structure and the number of divisions, plants or departments involved."

Definitions. After it has been determined which computer systems are validatable, each should be defined to describe its operation and function.

Computer System Validation Management. Those involved with the computer systems validation should be identified, along with their duties.

The Validation Protocol

"The easiest way to have consistency in the development of validation protocols is to outline the requirements as a checklist or a "fill in the blanks" document.

Documentation. *Since the validation protocol is documentation intensive, existing documents, reports, vendor manuals, etc. should be used. The development of protocol and the methodology used for validation should fit the existing management/committee structure whenever possible. Computer systems validation should not create a new documentation structure but rather pull together the necessary information for documentation and testing from that which already exists.*

Responsible People. *The first part should list the computer system and the person responsible for the validation process: for example, the department head or the user group, the responsible user. The other people responsible for the review, implementation, and approval of the protocol should be listed.*

Basis of Design. *A Basis of Design/Basis of Operation section should be included that can be used for both new and existing systems. For new systems, this section will provide clarity for purchase specifications. For an existing system it will document information that probably does not exist elsewhere. The main components of this section should include a narrative description of what the computer system is intended to do, a listing of requirements, the normal operating parameters (current memory requirements, number of ports currently used, etc.) and the absolute* *limits (maximum memory capacity, maximum number of ports, etc.). It may also be helpful to identify what the computer is not intended to do; this can prevent the system from being overloaded or misused.*

System Description. *The exact system that is either currently in operation or one that will be installed should be described. The hardware and all peripherals should be listed along with the applicable version of the operating software. The protocol should make provision for the documentation that both of these are certified at installation by the vendor using standard diagnostic programs. Applications software needs to be carefully documented and tested (verified) before it can be loaded into the operating hardware for operational testing and validation. The essential requirement for confidence in the software verification process is assured by the meticulous documentation of the specifications, planning, programming, testing, debugging and final "test data" verifying testing steps. Once the hardware/software information is collected, then all of the other pertinent data concerning the interaction with peripherals, equipment and instruments can be developed. If a system is used for material control, the materials should be adequately described (raw materials, package components, work in process and/or finished products) along with the methodology for switching to back up manual control.*

Hardware/Software.   *Diagrams of the hardware and hardware/software interactions are necessary for test plan development and auditing of the validation process. Unless your existing system is extremely well-controlled and documented, these diagrams will probably be the first complete identification of hardware/software interactions.*

Computer Room. *Computer rooms are usually constructed according to standard requirements of the major computer manufacturers. The details of the particular specifications for the computer room should be outlined for environmental conditions (temperature, humidity, line voltage and radio frequency interference). Consideration should be given to the differences in requirements for large computer rooms with multiple systems and for systems in production and laboratory areas. Each system should have a set of operating manuals and historical logs for: 1)hardware, 2)software, 3)critical events, 4)back-ups, and 5) maintenance/downtime. These logs should be maintained for periodic review and as an aid to change control. Appropriate consideration should also be given to computer rooms security.*

Customer Acceptance. *A new system installation and customer acceptance should be formally documented. Any changes to the system from the original specifications should be noted and all related documentation,* *including diagrams, should be updated. Existing systems should be documented as they are currently installed.*

SOPs. *SOPs are necessary for all aspects of the operation, maintenance, and change control of each system. They should be coordinated between the various departments to be sure all activities are covered. A grid of activities versus SOPs and responsible departments incorporated in the protocol is an effective double check on procedures.*

Training. *The system operators and users need to be trained. The responsible user should develop a training program in conjunction with the operating committee and the hardware/software suppliers, identify the operators/users and train them. This training should be documented in the form of a certificate for the individual and training status log for the system. All future training and system access must be appropriately authorized and documented since this is the cornerstone of internal system security and data integrity.*

Operational Testing. *The computer system should be operationally tested by the operators/users. Operational testing is the exercise of the verified applications software in the certified hardware/operations software system using test or simulated data. This can be accomplished in conjunction with the documentation of the operational qualification of the hardware/operating software during the validation testing.*

Validation Testing. *Validation testing is the exercise of the verified applications software in a certified hardware/operations software computer system using actual data in a simulated mode or on line concurrent testing with real time data. The requirements listed in the basis of design/basis of operation part of the protocol are the foundation for development of the test plan. The test plan need not be absolutely perfect; the validation process is an experimental study. If you find something wrong you have to figure out how to fix it. The software verification process should have eliminated the bugs but all possible circumstances cannot be foreseen. If the test plan is not complete, the problems and solutions can be described in the summary report; or, if they are serious problems, the solutions can be incorporated in a new validation test plan.*

Test Reports. *The essential data for the test reports that should be developed prior to testing are the system/module/subsystem being tested; the tests to be conducted; test references (if there are no literature references, the committee members responsible for the test design should be credited); test methodology, and acceptance criteria.*

Calibration. *Prior to the initiation of testing, all equipment, and instruments and interconnects should be calibrated.*

Testing. *Testing should be carried out according to the validation testing plan during realistic operating conditions.*

Protocol Summary. A summary of the protocol documentation including an analysis of the test results, the compliance audit of the system, and any system modifications should be submitted to the computer systems validation committee for their review and approval. It is recommended that the system not be used until final validation approval is received from the committee.

Audit Report. A report of independent audit of the computer validation process by an internal auditor (i.e. Quality Assurance) should be included with the summary report to management. The audit should compare the SOP and the initial parts of the protocol (what the system should do) with the test plan results (what the system actually does) and the summary report conclusions.

Permanent File. The original validation documentation should be maintained by Quality Control since they are the regulatory contact concerning validation."

These ideas of the SOP and the validation protocol, summarized in Figure 14-3, are not intended to be all-inclusive. They do, however, present an easy-to-comprehend method of beginning the task of computer system validation; and, as stated above, they point out that a lot of work will be required.

Validation Life Cycle

No examination of computer system validation should be considered complete without describing a concept which seems to be favored by both the FDA and the PMA — the *validation life cycle* (13,14,17). The

```
1. SOP
     - objective
     - descriptions
     - computer system validaton management

2. Validation Protocol
     - documentation            - responsible people
     - basis of design          - system description
     - hardware/software        - computer room
     - customer acceptance      - SOPs
     - training                 - operational testing
     - validation testing       - test reports
     - calibration              - testing
     - protocol summary         - audit report
     - permanent file
```

Figure 14-3. Summary — SOP and validation protocol.

validation life cycle closely resembles the traditional software development life cycle (20) (described in Chapter 11), which is as follows:

1. Requirements analysis
2. Specifications
3. Design
4. Programming
5. Testing
6. Integration testing
7. Deployment
8. Maintenance

In fact, the resemblance is so close that it must be from the development life cycle concept that the validation life cycle was developed.

In 1984, P.J. Motise (16) presented the "key elements of both hardware and software validation from the FDA's perspective." As we can see, these key elements easily map onto the development life cycle:

1. Defining tasks
2. Identifying limits
3. Testing
4. Preparing documentation
5. Revalidating

Then, in 1986, the PMA's report (17) outlined the validation program for a computer system as consisting of four sequential phases:

1. Prequalificaton — specification and design
2. Qualification — installation and operational checkout
3. Validation — testing
4. Ongoing evaluation

The validation concepts were considered using the life cycle approach, as shown in Figure 14-4. The components can be summarized (for new computer systems) as follows:

1. Definition
2. Develop Software
3. Testing
4. Integration testing
5. Acceptance
6. Ongoing use

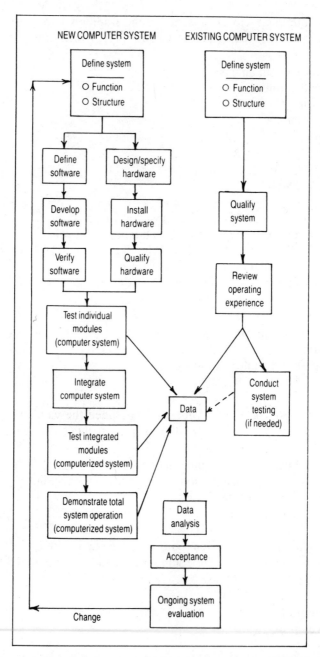

Figure 14-4. Validation life cycle. (PMA's Computer Systems Validation Committee. 1986. Validation concepts for computer systems used in the manufacture of drug products. *Pharm. Tech.* 10(5). p. 24-34)

In 1988, A.S. Clark (14) further refined the software life cycle approach to the following:

1. Development
2. Implementation
3. Testing
4. Maintenance
5. Documentation
6. Revalidation

Validation of Existing Computer Systems

At the *Pharm Tech* Conference of 1986, the FDA's P. Piasecki noted that the PMA's *Validation Concepts for Computer Systems Used in the Manufacture of Drug Products* (17) tended to "oversimplify the requirements for older systems that were installed and in operation before contemporary concepts regarding system validation were clearly recognized" (21). In 1987, the PMA responded when the PMA's Computer Systems Validation Committee member, James Agalloco, stated that "the validation of an existing computer system incorporates several distinct steps that closely resemble the corresponding steps taken to validate new systems". Agalloco presented the following steps:

1. System definition — summary of system functions.
2. System qualification — documentation of many items relating to system operation, including source code, drawings, and failure reports.
3. Testing the system — development of a validation protocol is the first step.
4. Related issues — security, change control, training and others.
5. Documentation — the validation report.
6. Ongoing system evaluation — upon approval of the validation report, the system should be treated like any other validatable system, new or old.

The main differences in the emphasis and application of these procedures to existing computer systems hinges on the predictable "inherent acceptability of the established system for its intended use" (21). Whether a system has been used to control a manufacturing process or to collect data from an instrument for a LIMS, the simple fact that it has produced acceptable results should be factored into the validation protocol, at least initially.

Why Do We Need to Validate Computer Systems?

Thus far in this chapter, we have examined the background of computer system validation concepts and pointed out some current views in this area. But some important questions still exist and need to be answered. Some of them are:

1. Why do we need to set up such procedures and extensive testing protocols?
2. Do we document computer system validation just because Federal regulations call for it?
3. What is the purpose of the regulatory requirements?

As stated above, the basic reason for validating a computer system is to make sure that it does what it is supposed to do. There are four fundamental, semi-independent components of computer systems which can cause failure or unexpected behavior of the system. These four components are hardware, software, the basic design of hardware and software, and environmental factors. Each of these components was mentioned above in one form or another, but an examination of each will help us strengthen our belief that computer system validation is for our own good, and not something we merely have to do.

Hardware

Computer hardware is becoming more and more reliable as each new generation of memory, input-output, CPU, and storage technologies debuts. In the not so distant past, to expect a medium-sized to large system to operate for as little as 30 days without a hardware failure was reasonable. Mean time between failures (MTBF) was once measured in days. Now, although many MTBFs are still listed in terms of days, they could easily be converted to months and even years.

In the early 1970s, the evolution of redundant and "hot backup" computer systems began in the process control industry. Many vendors subsequently found it advantageous to advertise redundant systems. Today redundancy is a standard feature of systems from almost every vendor. But although this feature is certainly prevalent throughout manufacturing and is certainly still demanded by process control engineers, redundancy is no longer the selling feature of control systems. This circumstance is due to a combination of standard redundancy features and a conscious, or sometimes unconscious, feeling that computer hardware is reliable.

Hardware reliability didn't happen overnight, or without high cost. Large scale integration technology advances have put more and more components closer together on chips, reducing cabling, connections, numbers of boards, and points of failure. Self-diagnosing chips and circuits are built into critical operating components, thus reducing overall component failure even when individual circuits fail.

Hardware failures are usually more easily diagnosed than those attributable to software. The use of hardware diagnostics was once an art. Field service engineers required long periods of time to isolate and solve complex problems. Now, diagnostic software, extensive support programs, and better-trained service engineers can routinely identify problem sources in much less time.

Despite all the good news about fewer hardware failures, longer MTBFs, and better service, the fact remains that hardware failures do put computer systems out of operation. Hardware failures can either shut down a system completely or cripple its operation, so that it must be shut down manually. Hardware failures must be expected and planned for. Such planning takes the following forms:

1. Purchase of redundant hardware components or systems for the most critical functions.
2. Preventive maintenance schedules.
3. Purchase of vendor service contracts.
4. In-house training and stocking of parts for hardware service for those providing their own maintenance.

Documentation of this planning, together with records of system failures, are required for computer system validation and should be an integral part of the validation protocol for each computer system.

Software

Behaviors — Unexpected and Gruesomely Sinister (**BUGS**). No matter how good we are at computer systems design and programming, our newly engineered and built systems will exhibit operational behaviors which are not expected. These unexpected behaviors are sometimes referred to as bugs. Why do bugs occur and what makes them an inevitable phenomenon? Let's face it, designing and programming complex software systems are not simple tasks. The systems analyst who designs a large, complex system must deal with many interrelationships and interactions among program modules, operating system constraints and parameters, multiuser-shared data and code concepts, nomenclature rules, file system dependencies, company expectations, customer expectations, hardware reliability, and even hardware speed. Systems must be engineered to withstand the elements of change, as described in Chapter 11. If the system development team consists of 10 systems analysts, then multiply the effect of these concerns by at least 10 — and perhaps even more, because inevitable differences in design ideas between two (or more) analysts will certainly require negotiation.

The complexity of the programming job is directly proportional to the complexity of the program or system being coded. Writing a single program consisting of 20 lines of code is not a complex task. Although the number is decreasing each year, many technical professionals routinely write their own short programs for solving daily problems that are both unique and repetitive. This number is decreasing because of the availability of software to interactively provide calculations, databases, graphics, and statistics. However, when new, large, complex computer systems are required, programming must be done. Programming such systems is a complex task. One of the primary skills required by a programmer is concentration. None of us may ever undertake a task requiring the concentration necessary to produce a complex computer system. Good programming techniques, documentation, and experience are essential in producing living, modifiable computer systems with reasonable and profitable life expectancies. The first two essentials, good programming techniques and documentation of the code, are learned in school by undergraduate systems analysts and associate degree programmers. But the third requirement, experience, comes from on-the-job training. Do we expect to staff every programming project with seasoned, experienced programmers? We would like to, but we don't always have that luxury.

Only through exhaustive testing and, unfortunately, operation can we hope to eliminate all the bugs in systems and gain enough confidence to trust these systems to produce reports from lab data, control the process, or forecast and manage inventory. Software development techniques and tools are evolving, along with all other aspects of computing. The time has come to expect software authors to deliver bug-free products, but we must still expect and plan for software errors. This planning takes the following forms:

1. Modular and integrated testing during development.
2. Purchase of vendor software support services; this is a good mechanism to use in reporting bugs.
3. Use of fourth-generation software development tools to minimize the need for new code.

4. Development of software that adheres to project management guidelines.

The only way to uncover all software bugs is through thorough testing of the code in actual operation. For new systems, testing of each module followed by testing after module integration is required. For existing systems, planned exercising of documented or believed software limits is useful in isolating potential problems. As with hardware, documentation of software testing should be part of the validation protocol.

Basic Design of Hardware and Software

Many system failures occur because the users expect something different from what the system was designed to do. The users request the system to perform at some level or in a manner that it is incapable of achieving. In these instances, the users don't know what the actual system performance, limits, or tolerances are. Having inaccurate expectations of system performance can be due to any of three reasons:

1. Improper or inadequate documentation/training.
2. Inadequate system design specifications.
3. A system design that differs from the specifications.

These three performance/expectation issues can be classified as basic design problems. Even in the case of improper or inadequate documentation/training, it is the system design that specified this requirement. Thus, if documentation is inadequate, it is the system design that is at fault. For purchased hardware and software, the design referred to here is the preselection specifications that are at fault, as described in Chapter 11. For in-house created systems, the design includes the preselection specifications, as well as the actual development and system integration.

Design and implementation of a protocol for system development and implementation, as described above, is the best way to avoid discrepancies between system design and performance. For existing and new systems alike, testing, testing, and testing is all that is required to identify these differences after development.

Environmental Factors

The condition of the electrical power feed to a computer system is one of the primary environmental factors which can easily lead to system failure or unexpected operation. Other significant factors are temperature, humidity, and electrical interference. Planning for these factors was covered in the discussion of the validation protocol in the section of "Computer Room."

Computer room conditions can be monitored and controlled by automatic, extremely sophisticated systems equipped with redundancy and even battery backup. It is totally inexcusable to allow the environment of a computer system to adversely affect the system's operation. However avoidable environmental failures are, they still happen. The primary reasons are unconditioned power, lack of battery backup, and air-conditioning failure. In addition, maintenance of the environmental control and monitoring systems, which is just as important as maintenance of the computer itself, is sometimes forgotten or neglected.

Planning for cooling failure is easy; simply provide dual air conditioners. Proper cooling capacity planning is extremely important. Normal operation may require both to be operational but each should be large enough to provide sufficient cooling for several hours in case one of the units fails. Cooling units consisting of both inside and outside pieces can be given an additional redundancy feature by allowing chilled or "city" water circulation, instead of the usual glycol, for times when the outside unit fails.

Power conditioners are readily available from many vendors. When they are used in conjunction with battery backup units, many electricity related problems can be solved.

Vendor Requirements

Generally, there is no problem in obtaining operation limits for hardware or software from vendors. Vendors of hardware systems will gladly provide environmental operating limits. Some vendors conduct on-site inspections prior to installation in order to identify problems or make suggestions to avoid problems. Vendor software specifications are usually supplied or readily available.

Problems related to vendor requirements and responsibilities in conjunction with computer system validation lie in understanding exactly what these requirements and responsibilities are. Should vendors be responsible for validation of the software they sell to customers with regulated applications?

The FDA Policy Guide 7132a.15 (23) suggests that careful scrutiny of vendor source code by users is desirable. The purpose is to determine "whether the purchased software meets acceptance specifications" (12). Chapman, Harris, Bluhm, and Errico (12) suggest, however, that a higher level of code review is more appropriate. They also list several references of useful techniques for software inspection, including the IEEE.

The PMA (17) states that the source code for nonapplication software which is purchased from a vendor, such as "operating systems, languages, screen design, automatic program generators, statistical packages, and report generators not specifically written for the user's system," is usually not available to the user. However, an agreement from the vendor should be obtained, perhaps contractually, that source code will be made available if the need arises.

It has been suggested (12) that the PMA CSVC's original attempt to separate software into application and nonapplication categories was oversimplified, and that there is an additional multicomponent level in between. The three layers of software are thus:

Level 1. Operating system, compilers, utilities.
Level 2. a. Executive source code — usually vendor supplied, such as run-time libraries.
        b. Configuration source code — command files or vendor-supplied control system utilities.
Level 3. Application-specific programs.

Eventually, the responsibility for validating commercial software must rest with its authors. Software is already being advertised as maintaining good laboratory practice standards. This definitely shows movement in the right direction. Customers must be able to depend on vendors to supply prevalidated software; otherwise, more of it may have to be written in-house.

LIMS and Validation Concepts

There are actually two levels of interest, related to LIMS, when considering validation concepts:

1. The LIMS itself, considered as a computer software system.
2. The data maintained by the LIMS.

For the LIMS itself, validation concepts relate to the development of the system and subsequent verification, after installation, that it is operating as intended. For the data maintained by the LIMS, validation concepts relate to regulatory and lab management standards involving data generation, test methods, data integrity, etc. In the sections below, we will consider these two levels separately as (1) LIMS — a computer software system, and (2) LIMS data.

LIMS — A Computer Software System

As noted above, when a computer system is involved in the manufacture or quality assurance of a product, it is a candidate for validation. Currently, LIMS are in place in every aspect of manufacturing from R&D to production quality control (24,26). It is hard to imagine an application for a LIMS which would disqualify it from validation. Of course, LIMS used in pharmaceutical, food product, and medical applications qualify without exception. Every computer system on which we depend to carry out our business, whether in the lab, in an office, or in a warehouse, should be periodically validated. Development of SOP and validation protocols for LIMS must be viewed as a part of the job. It is not an option.

There are certain tests which should be routinely performed on even an office PC, such as making sure that backup diskettes can be read on another machine to validate the disk drive's operation. The degree of testing required to ensure proper operation is proportional to the severity of the potential failure. If the office PC's disk fails and has to be replaced, the criticality of the new drive's ability to read the backup diskettes should determine the frequency of testing. For a LIMS which is used to report analytical data to a researcher who is working on new product development, testing may not be as critical as for a LIMS reporting analytical data to an operator on the manufacturing line. But even the LIMS reporting to the researcher should be tested frequently enough to ensure that it is functioning properly.

The requirements for LIMS computer system validation will vary among systems, depending on several factors, including:

1. The criticality of the system to daily operations.
2. The criticality of the system to manufacturing.
3. The criticality of the system to quality assurance.

As stated above, SOPs and validation protocols should not be considered optional for the LIMS. The success of ongoing validation depends on dedication to the belief that the benefit to the users will far outweigh the cost. If validation testing is done only to comply with some federal regulation, the point has been missed, and consequently the system users and even product quality will suffer in the long run.

The following sections consider computer system validation concepts as related to (1) the development of new LIMS and (2) application to existing systems.

Development of New LIMS

The validation protocol for a LIMS under development could easily be designed using the validation life cycle approach. Earlier, we discussed the life cycle as consisting of development, implementation, testing, maintenance, documentation, and revalidation. For a LIMS, the implementation, testing, and maintenance steps might require some unique talents generally not possessed by production programmers of computer systems. These rare talents include instrument interfacing, computer-to-computer links, and networking skills. However, for chemical and clinical laboratories which have been supported with in-house computer expertise for the past 20 years, computer people with these skills will probably be available.

A software development project, conducted with the goal of producing a system which is readily validatable, is possible. The odds of finding an individual who is able to produce such a system, and who also possesses the other skills required to build a LIMS, are remote. The computer support individuals with the necessary interfacing skills who work in laboratories will likely not have the training, ability, or inclination to produce a system using regimented system development techniques. The chances of putting a development team together which includes this combination of talents are also remote. Teams can be formed with in-house computer support personnel and in-house professional systems developers, but a successful LIMS product is not guaranteed. To expect a successful LIMS product which is designed for ease of validation is probably unreasonable.

As stated in Chapter 11, management of the LIMS development process should be under the control of the LIMS manager for several reasons, including the assurance that the system specifications are reflected in the final product. Hopefully, the LIMS manager will possess many of the skills needed to produce a successful LIMS, such as instrument interfacing. The manager is the key to the successful creation of a LIMS and to subsequent operational management; however, it is not reasonable to expect the manager to understand enough about software development techniques to ensure development of a readily validatable system.

One clear advantage that LIMS vendors have compared to industry's in-house development teams is that they are in a better position to maintain the necessary mix of expertise required to provide readily validatable software. First rate programmers and individuals with lab experience and knowledge can be assembled with the sole purpose of producing first rate, readily validatable LIMS software. Of course, in-house program development could also accomplish this task, but it is not likely to happen. And even if it did, what about continuing support? Continuing support means constant cross-training. What about new versions with bug fixes and new features? How long will all the initial features be sufficient? To what extent can companies afford to maintain an in-house written package when, after a period of time, better software becomes commercially available? The LIMS vendors, whose business it is to make their product better than their competitors', have the resources and incentive to worry about new features, bug fixes, and continuing support. It is their business to maintain the assemblage of specialized individuals required to produce and enhance LIMS software, especially when the requirement is complicated with system validation concerns.

Existing LIMS

The validation of existing LIMS should follow the outline presented above for existing systems, which consists of system definition, system qualification, testing the system, related issues, documentation, and on-going system evaluation. It may initially appear that testing and ongoing evaluation the same; however, there are some differences, the primary one should be noted before continuing. The purpose of testing is to make sure that the existing system is currently operating as intended. The purpose of ongoing evaluation is the same for any system, old or new; to ensure that it continues to operate as intended.

Application of the steps for validation of existing systems to LIMS is not difficult, but it requires a lot of work and, again, dedication to the belief that the benefit provided to the system users will far outweigh the cost. Figure 14-5 presents some suggestions for applying the existing systems validation steps to LIMS. These suggestions are definitely not all inclusive. They are presented as examples of what might be expected for each of the steps. The composite plan presented may be adequate for some LIMS but for only a subset of the whole for others.

LIMS Data

Assuming that we can build or find a LIMS which meets our computer system validation requirements, the capability provided by the LIMS must comply with good laboratory practice standards. "Fortunately, many of the requirements of such standards are very amenable to proper automation, greatly reducing the cost and effort of compliance" (28).

1. **System Definition** – Describe the functions performed
   by the LIMS such as sample LOGIN and RECEIVE. Describe
   the use of WORKSHEETS and COLLECTION LISTS. Indicate how
   reports are issued. The use LIMS supervisory functions
   such as BACKLOG, ARCHIVE, TURNAROUND TIME should be
   outlined.
2. **System Qualificaton** – Use drawings to illustrate data flow
   within analytical laboratories showing how data enters and
   exits the lab. When raw data is obtained followed by
   calculations to produce results, the calculations should
   be explained. References to the location of source code
   should be provided. Obtaining written agreement to provide
   source code if needed should be obtained from the vendor
   when using a commercial package. System usage logs,
   including failure reports, should be kept.
3. **Testing the system** – The purpose of this step is to
   validate that the system is performing as intended.
   Detailed scrutiny should be done on all aspects of the
   system should be performed. Development of a validation
   protocol is the first step. Every aspect of the system
   including the data base design, capacity, and content
   should be checked. All enhancement projects should be
   postponed until all parts of the existing system are
   examined.
4. **Related issues** – The method for determining which users
   have access to what functions should be described. All
   system security policies should be cited. Training
   guidelines should be presented along with training course
   outlines.
5. **Documentation** – The definitions, qualificatons, and
   listings should be assembled in the form of a report and
   submitted to management for their approval. This report
   is the validation report. It should be updated regularly
   in accordance with the operating procedure for the system.
6. **ONGOING system evaluation** – The standard operating
   procedure for the LIMS should define the validation
   protocol to be used for ongoing system evaluation. Testing
   should include procedures done daily to insure integrity of
   the system. Other procedures which might require system
   down time, such as verifying backup procedures, would
   probably not be scheduled daily, but should be done
   regularly.

Figure 14-5. Validation procedure for existing LIMS.

Most commercial LIMS systems address these standards with design
and performance features. Figure 14-6 summarizes the compliance features offered by the Beckman CALS Lab Manager System (28). These
features are described below as examples of what might be found in
commercial systems and what should be designed into in-house systems.

   GLP compliance features, such as those for the Beckman CALS Lab
Manager system, are also found in the other commercial LIMS. Features
such as these guarantee the accuracy of the data and information flowing
into and out of the LIMS. Without such guarantees, it would be understandably difficult to have faith in LIMS processes, which greatly reduce
paper methods of operation.

Security — The capability to enable or disable LIMS features to users as their need demands.

Audit Trail — Entry and modification of test results as well as revision of test methods, are automatically stamped with the time, date, and ID of the LIMS user.

Document Control — Reports include time and date of generation and are labeled as "original," "preliminary," or "duplicate."

Data Archiving and Recall — All data is archived. Recalled data is so marked.

Data Indexing and Retrieval — Data may normally be retrieved by database key, but can also be retrieved by values of any field.

Instrument Calibration and Maintenance — Automatic scheduling of instruments for calibration and maintenance with accumulation of maintenance and usage history.

Time, Date and User ID Stamp — All test results are automatically stamped with current time, date, and user ID.

Data Validation — Validation of test results against preset limits, flagging values which are out of limits, generation of exception reports, and manual verification of tests results if desired.

System Validation — Validation programs are supplied with the system to verify correct database structure.

Automatic Database Verification — Data integrity is assured even through system disasters by the unique safegard technique of "mirroring" the active database automatically. When mirror images are placed on two separate disk drives, the probability of losing more than a single transaction due to hardware or power failure is infinitesimally small.

Source Code — Source code is available upon execution of the appropriate non-disclosure agreements.

Documentation — System operation, as well as tests, reports, procedures, and security classes are completely documented.

Management Oversight — Specifications, limits, methods, and report formats are always current and are simultaneously updated for all users.

Figure 14-6. Beckman CALS lab manager GLP/GMP compliance features. (Beckman Instruments, Inc. Laboratory. *Information Management and Data Acquisition System*. Waldwick, N.J. p. 5-27)

A Hidden Benefit of Computer Systems Validation

Software vendors compete by providing better features than their competitors. When one vendor develops a novel feature, a similar one will show up in competitors' products. For purchased software, bug fixes and new features are obtained in new version releases. Thus, ongoing support in terms of bug fixes and new features are expected with purchased software support for commercial software.

There is a benefit, perhaps hidden, in the application of validation concepts to in-house developed computer systems, including LIMS. The benefit is found in the area of ongoing support for computer software systems. Ongoing support for in-house developed systems is often more expensive than support for purchased systems, and LIMS is no exception. The basic reason for the additional expense is quite complicated. In general, ongoing support for in-house developed systems decreases with time. After the initial development project, the amount of resources given to supporting the system is usually never adequate. New features are not developed as needed, and bugs are not fixed as they are found. The result is a system which is underutilized and/or which is not used efficiently. The combination of these two problems represents a tremendous expense to companies. When the system's users complain enough or when system usage falls sufficiently, some effort is made to solve the immediate problems, and the cycle begins again.

Conformance to a validation protocol will itself go a long way toward ensuring that proper ongoing support for the system and its users will be provided. Ongoing validation is part of the validation protocol. It is in the"Ongoing Validation" section of the protocol that one should build in guarantees that bugs are being fixed as found and that new features are being added as needed.

Summary

In this chapter, we have seen that the purpose of computer system validation is to ensure that a system does what it is supposed to do in a reliable manner. The target of federal GLP compliance guidelines for computer systems was, originally, limited to process control systems involved in pharmaceutical manufacturing. Since the early 1980s, any list of validatable computer systems has included systems involved in the quality assurance of any product.

"Computer systems validation is not a new, magic formula. The techniques are the same ones used in any structured approach to project management" (11). The validation life cycle approach to computer systems validation closely aligns with software development life cycles which have existed since the 1960s. Maintaining SOPs which include validation protocols for our computer systems will enable users to guarantee that systems are performing in the manner in which they were intended.

The application of validation procedures to LIMS is very simple. A six-step procedure for an existing LIMS is as follows:

1. System definition
2. System qualification
3. Testing the system
4. Related issues
5. Documentation
6. Ongoing system evaluation

This procedure is a means to begin applying validation concepts to LIMS. It is suggested as a place to start. The size and scope of the project will determine how much work needs to be done in each step.

Chapter 15

Justification for a LIMS

Before describing the best way to justify a LIMS installation, this chapter discusses the pitfalls and drawbacks associated with installing a LIMS. Whether one is a lab manager, production manager, lab analyst, director of research, or vice president, one must understand the problems which must be solved before a LIMS can be successful. Justification, selling the idea of a LIMS, installation, maintenance, and growth of a LIMS are not easy. The problems which exist are not technological; they are human. "What makes the introduction and evolution of [information technology (IT)] so challenging is that, in many of its applications, success comes only when people have changed their thinking process. Hence we will refer to it as *intellectual technology*. Without this concomitant change in thinking, we too frequently have a technical success but an administrative failure" (60).

By first examining the problems associated with a LIMS, we will be better able to comprehend the reasons for using a LIMS in an analytical laboratory environment.

Pitfall Experience

When beginning a project which will result in reaching some goal, it is always beneficial to have advance warning of possible pitfalls which may be encountered along the way. This is true for every project we undertake. Some examples are:

An automobile trip — Advance knowledge of shortcuts, the locations of road work, rush hour bottlenecks, and good places to stop for food and sleep can not only save travel time but can dramatically reduce tension and frustration.

A backyard barbecue party — Knowing the weather forecast, how many to cook for, the quantity of gas remaining in the grill, and whether to expect any vegetarians can mean the difference between a successful party and a failure.

Installation of computer hardware — Delays are inevitable if prior knowledge of floor space dimensions, electrical and air conditioning maximum loads, plug/receptacle sizes, and cable length requirements are not known in advance.

Considering example 3, the installation of computer hardware, we would expect the hardware vendor to be able (and always willing) to help minimize the effects of possible pitfalls. In many cases, of course, installation either comes with the hardware or is purchased. In these instances, although someone else is worrying about the pitfalls, they can still cause delay — but the probability of delay is less. What we actually pay for when we purchase installation of computer equipment is the experience of the vendor in dealing with the possible pitfalls. And *experience* is the key word.

The purchase of experience is insurance against the effects of pitfalls which are unknown. For many projects and undertakings, we may be able to purchase "pitfall experience"; however, for many others, such as examples 1 and 2 above, the experience will have to be personal or will be hard to acquire.

Pitfalls of a LIMS Installation

Many times when we begin a project such as the installation of a LIMS, we either don't recognize that there may be pitfalls or we tend to ignore them. By recognizing that there are pitfalls and even possible drawbacks to a LIMS installation, trying to learn what they are, and being prepared to meet them head on, the probability of project success is greatly enhanced. Installation times can be greatly reduced by understanding and preparing for as many pitfalls as can be identified.

The following sections describe some of the factors involved which complicate and add to the difficulty of installing a LIMS in an exiting laboratory. These factors, summarized in Figure 15-1, are the pitfalls and drawbacks of a LIMS installation.

LIMS Are Not Cheap

The cost of a commercial LIMS, including both hardware and software, ranges from $20,000 to $300,000 for a stand-alone system. On the low end are PC-based systems consisting of one PC, usually an IBM PC or a compatible model. On the high end are large, multiuser minicomputer-based systems. The single PC-based system is intended for a relatively

1. LIMS are not cheap
   - impact on existing computer system
2. Hard to justify LIMS on clerical or effort savings
3. LIMS don't come with an on button (30)
4. Installing a LIMS has possible drawbacks (31) and risks
   which are:
   a. cost overruns owing to underestimated development
      times
   b. delays in implementation
   c. lab disruption
   d. reduced moral
   e. lower lab efficiency
   f. disruption of service to customers

Figure 15-1. Pitfalls and drawbacks of installing LIMS.

small laboratory with a small sample count, a small requirement for instrument interfacing, and few customers. The large minicomputer-based system is, of course, just the opposite. It is designed for a large number of concurrent users, generally several dozen.

The perception of expense is also relative. Many laboratories considering low-end products will believe that $20,000 is too high, while others will find this price reasonable for the performance delivered. The same is true for larger laboratories considering high-end systems. Some will believe that $300,000 is too high, while others will find it reasonable.

The performance required of a LIMS, such as the number of concurrent users, number of samples processed, size of the database, etc., will certainly play a large part in determining its cost. The larger the scope of the LIMS, the larger the host machine requirement, and the higher the cost. (A mechanism for determining system requirements is presented in Chapter 11.) If an existing computer system is available which could be used as the LIMS host, the initial cost of getting started with a LIMS is greatly reduced. A laboratory planning to purchase LIMS software for a large minicomputer can expect to pay around $100,000 for the software plus installation. LIMS which are priced in this range, installed on a large computer, are capable of handling very large projects.

LIMS Installation Has an Impact on an Existing Computer System

Installation of a LIMS on an existing computer system will, of course, have some impact on the other users and applications of the system. A LIMS is not a CPU-intensive application. It is a typical database application which involves an input/output-intensive requirement. However, the effect on other users of the system, whether using the LIMS or some other application, will be the same. Applications which are highly input/output intensive can and do cause a real slow down of the system.

Most large computer systems can be operated and/or upgraded to reduce the effects of input/output-intensive applications. High-speed disk drives can be added or purchased to replace older, slower models. Databases can be placed on one or more disk drives which separate them from system utilities and other applications. Intelligent disk controllers can be purchased to optimize and speed disk access. Even operating system parameters can be adjusted to favor input/output-intensive applications at the expense of other applications. As expected, these types of hardware enhancements aren't cheap. Likewise, adjustments of parameters to make the LIMS run faster will make other applications run slower and thus involve some cost.

There is a cost associated with putting the LIMS on an existing system. This arrangement will certainly appear to reduce the initial cost of getting started. But, unfortunately, there is no magic formula to determine the cost to the other users of the system. Disk capacity may not have to be purchased to accommodate the initial installation, but the cost of the disk storage requirement should certainly be considered. Enlarging other applications may not be possible after the LIMS is installed due to the additional number of concurrent users added by the LIMS. Other applications may have to be moved to other systems to make room for the LIMS. The percentage of system resources required for the LIMS must be estimated by the system manager and the LIMS manager with the help of the vendor.

Concerns other than direct cost- and capacity-related issues also exist when considering a LIMS installation on an existing computer system. Ownership and management of the system must also be considered. Does the system belong to the lab or to the management information system (MIS) department? If the lab is to support the LIMS, it may not be desirable to install it on a system owned and managed by MIS. Also, reliability of the LIMS host should always be of primary concern. New computers are generally more reliable than old ones, although a substantial maintenance program must be in effect for either.

LIMS Are Hard to Justify on a Clerical or Effort Savings Basis

Obviously, the ideal way to justify an expense or capital expenditure is by the elimination of effort. Effort savings come in several forms:

- Reduction in personnel
- Eliminating the need for additional personnel
- Performing some function faster, allowing that function to be performed with greater frequency
- Clerical savings, which include reduction of paperwork

Reduction in existing personnel will seldom, if ever, be made possible by the installation of a LIMS. Generally, laboratory managers who are looking for ways to reduce staff must also look for services which can be discontinued. If the need for a service being provided by a laboratory decreases or disappears, then staff reductions become desirable.

A problem which is perhaps more representative of most laboratories is how to accomplish more with existing personnel. This problem is approached by increasing efficiency. Increasing efficiency can easily eliminate the need for additional personnel to accomplish a given performance goal. The performance level of any laboratory is based on the resources available, both human and equipment, and the efficiency with which they operate. A LIMS allows the human resources to perform more efficiently, thus reducing the need for additional personnel. This is accomplished by enabling lab tasks to be performed more efficiently, including a reduction in clerical demand. The LIMS takes care of issuing reports, archiving the data, producing control charts, checking test limits, and many other things. Increasing the lab's output also means increasing the types of functions that a LIMS can do more efficiently than humans. Certainly, additional staff can be added to increase performance, but probably at a higher cost than that of adding a LIMS. Still, these kinds of savings are hard to quantify and often hard to sell to management.

In Chapter 1 we noted that a LIMS, properly implemented, can help to control the information management process in laboratories in order to get the most out of the data. This type of benefit does not seem to relate directly to clerical or effort savings. But, when considered in terms of increasing laboratory efficiency, it falls neatly into place. To bring the process of laboratory information management under control, what is needed? One could certainly begin by applying statistical process control (SPC) methods to instrumentation. Control charting of standard samples to aid in verification of results is a tool that most laboratories have probably been using for a long time. But are all lab methods and instruments being managed in this fashion?

Managing laboratory inputs and outputs using SPC methods is also desirable. The number of samples entering the lab for a particular test must be measured for predictive purposes to facilitate resource allocation. In addition, turnaround times and backlogs are typical management tools which deal with lab inputs and outputs. How does increasing laboratory performance affect these types of information management? It requires more work. Applying SPC methods to tests, instruments, and sample counts takes time. A LIMS can perform the extra work without adding additional staff. A LIMS may be hard to justify by simply saying that its use will reduce effort. The use of a LIMS will allow a smaller staff to accomplish more, and thus increase efficiency.

In Chapter 1, we also noted that a LIMS can help laboratories withstand the multitude of changes to which they are subjected. Being able to withstand change is key to the success and profitable operation of a lab. Change occurs continuously. Without a process in place to monitor change, a lab will not be able to adapt correctly. For example, reacting too quickly or too slowly to changes in requests for analysis could result in too many or too few resources. A LIMS can easily monitor numbers of samples and test requests. Human effort could certainly be used to perform this type of monitoring, but definitely at a higher cost.

LIMS Don't Come with an On Button

Some effort is required to install and set up a LIMS before it can begin to work. User accounts, test methods, and other information must be supplied to the LIMS before it can be used, as described in Chapter 9. The amount of initial setup required will depend on the scope of the project. The scope takes into account the size and complexity of the LIMS, as described in Chapter 11. The more users and test methods to be included in the LIMS environment, the more setup is required. These types of setup, although required, are facilitated by setup screens provided by the LIMS.

Most LIMS can be both tailored and customized. The difference between these two concepts is described in Chapter 4. The purpose of both is the same: to mold and enhance the LIMS in order to either increase its performance or to blend it more closely into lab operations. Customization is required to interface instruments and to automate other procedures, such as producing control charts automatically. We noted earlier that the amount of benefit which might be derived from a LIMS is directly related to how well the system is managed. The amount of benefit is also related to how well the system blends in with lab operation. Tailoring and customization are the means by which the LIMS can be made to perform in such a manner as to achieve the most benefit. Much of the tailoring of a LIMS can be accomplished during installation and setup. Customization, by contrast, can continue indefinitely, for as long as the LIMS is used. Customization is required to interface new instruments and to respond to customer requests. These needs will continue for as long as the LIMS is used. Staffing to provide customization support must be considered in the cost of operating the LIMS.

As we described in Chapter 11, there should be a period of intense support followed by a period of continuing support. The LIMS support team should be larger during the intense support period. During the continuing support period, the support team should consist of two to four persons for a large LIMS. Smaller systems can thrive with a one-

or two-person team during the continuing support period. During the intense support period, the LIMS team should consist of four to six, or even more persons depending on the scope of the project. Again, staffing to provide this support must not be forgotten or ignored when considering a LIMS installation.

Chapter 13 discusses training for LIMS users. The benefit potential of a LIMS is also related to how well the users are trained in its operation. Training is expensive. The time required to design the training courses, when done in house, must be considered. The time required by the instructors, as well as that of the trainees, is substantial when all users are considered. Assuming 200 users, each trained on LIMS operation for 4 hours, plus the instructor's time, totals approximately 1000 hours invested in training.

Thus, the laboratory doesn't just buy a LIMS, install it, and turn it on. There are setup, customization, training, and support requirements. Solutions to any of these requirements can be purchased (or hired) either from the LIMS vendors or from a growing LIMS consultant/contractor base. The cost to provide these functions should be carefully examined with the LIMS vendor. The vendor can provide customizations for specific projects, perhaps less expensively than doing the project in-house. The vendor can be brought on site for training to save lengthy course development expense. However these requirements are provided, it is very important to realize at the onset, during initial requirements evaluation whenever possible, that there are other substantial expenses involved. These expenses can far surpass that of the initial purchase.

Possible Drawbacks

The above LIMS implementation pitfalls, although extremely important, encompass some fairly vague concepts such as expense and justification. A second set of possible pitfalls is far more tangible and perhaps easier to comprehend. These pitfalls are the ones dealt with on a day-to-day basis. We will call them drawbacks. They consist of cost overruns, delays, lab disruption and reduced morale, lower lab efficiency, and disruption of service to customers. These drawbacks, like the other pitfalls, are potential problems, not imminent problems.

There is one categorical difference between the pitfalls and the drawbacks, however, which deals with the certainty of their occurrence. The pitfalls described above relate to expense and justification. Their effect can be minimized by being prepared for them and meeting them head on, as stated above. They have to be dealt with in one form or another, sooner or later — and the sooner the better. As for the drawbacks, proper management of the LIMS project can all but eliminate them. As we will see, the possible drawbacks are countered with planning, implementation rate, training, and encouragement.

Cost Overruns.   A cost overrun for a LIMS implementation project is due to underestimating the installation and development times. As we saw in Chapter 11, the time from the beginning of the preinstallation planning period to the end of the intense support period, may be approximately 4 years for a large LIMS. Such LIMS includes the following minimum components:

Over 100 active test methods
Over 200 active users
Over 1000 samples per week
Various automated instrumentation

A LIMS doesn't come with an on button. A lot of effort is needed to integrate all the methods, users, samples, and instrumentation with the information relating to each. The LIMS is merely a tool to facilitate the integration. It is not a magic software/hardware black box. Of course, time requirements will vary dramatically, depending on the size of the LIMS team. A LIMS which meets these minimum scope measurements would require approximately 4 years for a relatively small team of two to three very good individuals — about eight effort years.

The rate of implementation of the LIMS project must be managed. To implement the project in 1 year would seemingly require an eight-person team (for a project with a minimum scope, as measured above), but not necessarily. It should be staffed in the beginning with two to three very good, full time, individuals (again, depending on the scope), rather than overstaffed. After about 6 months, an additional one to two persons can be added to the team. Some tasks must be done serially. Also, the LIMS team will learn as they implement and improve with time.

Implementation effort should be estimated on the high side. It is always better to overestimate effort requirements and subsequently to require less. The fact remains that LIMS are not cheap. A cost overrun is a burden on any project. Poorly implemented projects, which have overrun burdens, are candidates for failure.

Implementation Delays.   Implementation delays for a LIMS project are, for the most part, the same as those for any small-team project. Individuals have unique responsibilities that are not duplicated within the team. If one individual is not able to accomplish her or his projects on schedule, for whatever reason, the whole project will suffer. Illness, vacation, or demands of the job can cause delays. For example (a true case), severe delays were caused in a large LIMS implementation because the LIMS manager became involved with communications and system management functions, since there was no one else to handle them. These functions were also important and had to be done. As a result, the LIMS project suffered.

In early project stages, especially during product evaluations, delays are frequent because of travel and other logistic problems related to viewing products from many different vendors. In later stages, solving morale and disruption problems (described below) will require extra time and will result in LIMS implementation delays.

Instrument-to-computer/LIMS interfacing is a complex concept which requires highly talented individuals capable of visualizing the intricacies of the connections and then transferring them to code. Many details must be dealt with, and there are many opportunities for delay. Experience is the only weapon against delays in this area.

As the LIMS implementation project progresses, new projects will be identified. As the LIMS users become comfortable with the system and learn its capabilities, they will have many good suggestions for improvements. Some of the new ideas for projects will appear more useful than others and rise quickly to the top of the project list. One must be very careful in managing this type of project scheduling. The benefits of one project may clearly outweigh those of another, but if it means rescheduling the less worthy project or perhaps missing its target date, then a very careful evaluation of the projects must be done. Are there customers waiting for the less beneficial project? Have promises been made concerning a target date? If someone has been promised that a new method will be in place by a certain date, then it may be better to meet that date than to schedule another project with higher benefit potential in front of it. The worst thing that can happen during a LIMS installation is to alienate users. If this could possibly happen, the new project should be scheduled after the one already scheduled. It will pay off in the long run because no delay will be introduced into the process.

Lab Disruption and Reduced Moral.   Interruption or perturbation of sample and/or information flow through an analytical laboratory can cause disruption. For example, if the main instrument is out of service for some reason, backlogs rise. And so do anxieties. If analytical results are used to control a process, delay of the results report, for whatever reason, creates pressure from both internal and external lab sources.

Occasional short-lived periods of decreased throughput and below normal output quality can occur in any analytical laboratory. A symptom of disruption in an analytical laboratory is that laboratory processes which normally run well within control limits shift to operating clearly out of control and do not snap back within a very short period of time. The bottom line is that throughput and output quality suffer.

Adjustments in laboratory processes are usually implemented either to improve the quality of the lab's output, to decrease sample turnaround time, or to increase the number of samples which can be processed in a given amount of time. Sometimes when adjustments are made, efficiency or sample numbers may decrease for a period of time. These effects are usually caused by a learning curve brought about by new instrumentation, new methods, new sample types, etc. Experienced lab managers will anticipate learning curves and plan steps to avoid possible disruption. Overtime scheduled in advance, ample training time scheduled in advance, forewarning lab analysts and technicians of process adjustments and expected learning curves, and encouragement are helpful to those dealing with new involvements in the lab.

The installation of a LIMS in a laboratory (or group of laboratories) brings a set of adjustments to laboratory processes. The potential for disruption is present. In fact, this type of process adjustment often creates more disruption than others. The inclusion of a new set of computer programs in the lab's processes will act as a clouding agent. From the viewpoint of lab members, the lab processes which were clear and well understood will become unfamiliar and have an air of uncertainty subsequent to the LIMS installation. Of course, the processes will become clear again after a period of use. Also, proper training will help lessen the clouding affect. The more the lab members know about the LIMS before they are expected to use it and depend on it, the less disruption will occur.

A prime cause of disruption is the reduction of morale in one or more lab members. Some of the lab members will favor using the LIMS, and others won't. If people feel that the LIMS is being forced on them without their consent, or feel that the training has been inadequate, then morale suffers, disruption is imminent, and the LIMS will incur unnecessary blame. Everyone is reluctant to change — some more than others. We all like to know what faces us and how to handle it, especially on the job. Many of us don't like challenges. We'd rather have things stay the same. If fact, some individuals cannot handle change. When change occurs, morale suffers. When the LIMS is causing the change, it will get the blame for the disruption caused by the decrease in morale.

Many lab analysts do not deal with concerns external to their own laboratory. Through no fault of their own, they do not see the interrelationships between laboratory units in enough detail to perceive the "big picture." As a consequence, if a new LIMS is not far better than the old sample handling methods, it will receive bad publicity. If it doesn't make their job easier enough to offset the change in day-to-day operations, it may be rejected. If the LIMS takes a little longer to use per sample than the old methods, again, it may be rejected by the analysts. It may not be clear to lab analysts why getting test results back a day sooner to the sample submitter is good for the company and far offsets the inconvenience they may have to live with until they become familiar with the new LIMS. Lab analysts and even some lab managers do not know the value of the information that they are producing.

It is never desirable to force the implementation of a LIMS. If the users do not understand the value of information management and are not sold on using the LIMS, morale will suffer and disruptions will occur. The LIMS users must be trained and educated about the value of laboratory information and why it must be managed to derive all of its potential benefit. An educational program designed to show information as a company asset and stress its value should be required for all laboratory members.

Lower Lab Efficiency.   Although application of a LIMS may be good for the organization as a whole, it may actually reduce efficiencies in some areas. For analytical tests which cannot be automated, the need to enter test results at a terminal may require more time than writing the results on a piece of paper. Thus, efficiency appears to be hurt and the potential for morale problems is high. Even for automated methods, in the beginning there will most likely be an additional time requirement to use the LIMS as the lab shifts from the old methods. At a certain time, both the old and new methods may be in simultaneous use. Some samples will arrive in the lab submitted the old way, and some will arrive submitted on LIMS.

The beginning of the LIMS implementation, as it is first installed in a new area, is the most critical time for the project. Opinions as to its usefulness will be made which will be hard to change later. If situations such as simultaneous use of both the old and new systems can be minimized, implementation will be much easier and will happen faster.

The LIMS implementation team must always use its imagination to find ways of making the LIMS attractive or even transparent to its users. But no matter how good the LIMS team is, there will be instances where using LIMS will require more effort than the methods it is replacing. Again, the way to manage the problems associated with this circumstance is to educate lab members as to the value of the information and the value of capturing it in an information management system.

Disruption of Service to Customers.   During periods of disruption in the lab, the quantity and quality of service to the lab's customers will suffer.

For a lab that bills for its services, disruption results in decreased revenue. For organizations with internal customers, whether they are billed or not, service disruptions result in questions and pressure from management. All of the potential pitfalls and drawbacks to a LIMS implementation project can result in disruption of service to customers. This is the primary reason for trying to minimize the effects of the pitfalls and drawbacks.

Turnaround times, backlogs, and sample counts should be monitored very closely during the LIMS implementation. Lab customers who are internal to the organization should be kept informed of progress during the LIMS implementation and should be warned that potential disruptions are possible.

Implementing a LIMS Is a Culture Change

The concept of culture change in business is related to exhibiting different behavior over time. It is also related to mental adaptation to a set of beliefs which account for the behavior. There have been several worldwide culture changes in the laboratory over the past two decades. An obvious one is the use of computing technology. Electronics built with computer circuitry are included in all electronic laboratory instruments. Multipurpose computing is now a requirement in laboratories for data processing, calculations, and data presentation by graphs, charts, and word processing. Computing technology is now found in nearly every analytical and physical testing laboratory. It is an accepted tool for helping workers to perform job functions. The applicability of a PC to laboratory operations is no longer questioned. The old timers who questioned the benefit of computing in laboratories some 10 years ago, are now gone — and they never changed their beliefs. The old timers of today, who will be gone 10 years from now, are changing their beliefs. They are not only accepting the new technology but are staunchly supporting it. Newcomers in labs today are growing up with computing technology. Thus, a culture change has occurred.

The foundation for the computing culture change was laid 15 to 20 years ago. Laboratory newcomers in that period saw the change coming and probably played a role in making it a reality. The application of LIMS in our laboratories is a culture change. It will take time for beliefs to change, which will affect behaviors. But it is happening. For example, newcomers to labs now have no belief that laboratory notebooks are sacred, as many did in the past. Instead, they are asking, "Why can't I keep data and results on the computer?" In fact, using a computer to maintain lab records is becoming as natural as using a notebook. Within 5 years, it will be the standard method.

We are now in the period where the old-timers currently in our labs are ready to adopt the new LIMS technology. Those who were incapable of believing that LIMS will be the next culture are now gone. Those who have already adapted computing technology can see the benefits of automated computer methods of data and information handling. Newcomers to labs now expect to use computer systems to enable them to perform more efficiently. The culture change has begun.

Installing a LIMS Should Be a Leadership Process

In Chapter 4 we discussed the notion of the LIMS champion, someone who is responsible for plowing the ground initially and planting the initial LIMS seeds, which subsequently lead to the LIMS installation (the harvest). No matter how well the LIMS implementation is managed, however, some individuals will find reasons to object and will be unwilling to support the project; unfortunately, there may even arise the LIMS antichampion. The delays, disruption, reduced morale, lower efficiency, and reduced service to customers will be cited as evidence that the LIMS is a waste of time and money. "Most LIMS horror stories are characterized by laboratory personnel who were ignored or disinterested" (34). The antichampion(s) has been alienated for some reason or enjoys the attention gained from assuming the negative role. Of course, an antichampion may not emerge, but when he or she does, this is the worst thing that can happen. At best, there will be passive resistance by those who are unwilling to help the project but are not outspoken about it.

Should a battle be waged against the negative forces? Will they go away if left alone? What is the best method of dealing with them? In business, there are several means of persuading others to see things differently and behave differently. Some of them are economic, battling it out, political, supervisory rank order, and leadership. Each will be briefly described.

Economic Methods.   Cost reductions, effort savings, material savings, etc., are economic measures for justification of projects, expenditures, personnel requisitions, and so on. Justifications based on economics are less time consuming to explain because they are easier to understand. Unfortunately, the economics of many projects related to long term investment and culture change are hard to visualize.

Battling It Out.   When peers are faced with opposing views, many times a battle ensues. Most of the time, the opponents hope that the terms of battle will be friendly and that a clear winner will emerge. But how often does just the opposite occur? Enemies are made, and the decisions are never black and white and clear-cut. Battles occur when the economics are uncertain or about the same for each side.

Political Methods.   Many times, games are played to accomplish a purpose, obtain support, and obtain approval. The prime example of such a game is "you scratch my back and I'll scratch yours." These games are played by individuals who enjoy working this way and who are good at it. Many problems are solved by political maneuvers and they are a fact of life, even in the laboratory. But unfortunately, some individuals have absolutely no success in dealing in this manner. Also, when it comes to impressing a large number of individuals, political means often fall short.

Supervisory Rank Order.   If a supervisor wants an employee to behave in a certain manner, the supervisor can simply instruct the employee on the desired behavior and everything will be okay. Right? We all know better. Yes, the employee may behave the way the supervisor wants this time, but what about next time? How will this action be perceived by others?

Leadership.   Influencing behavior by being a leader in demonstrating the desired behavior is a powerful management tool. If a manager desires a certain behavior from employees, the first place to start is with her or his own behavior and then offer positive reinforcement for those who follow. Managing by example requires commitment to the cause. It takes time to learn enough about a project to gain commitment to its success in order to become the leader. Positive reinforcement is often hard for some managers to deliver. Thus, influencing behavior by exercising leadership is too often underrated, underestimated, and underused.

It is possible to justify a LIMS with a small scope using economic arguments. Sometimes a LIMS can return results sufficiently faster than manual methods to justify the expense. Sometimes the LIMS can provide a platform for automation and data management sufficient enough to justify the expense. Sometimes the value of the data integrity provided by LIMS in regulated environments justifies the expense. However, the justification of a LIMS should not be based on economic measures. Investment in a LIMS is an investment in the future. Electronic data management is a reality. Simply put, it is more efficient than manual methods because it provides capabilities that would be unaffordable if done manually. Electronic information management is also a reality. It is a new technology in the laboratory environment. It has grown since the early 1980s, and will continue to evolve and define new levels of laboratory efficiency and information values.

The implementation of any strategy is a means to remain competitive in the future. The investment in a LIMS is the implementation of a strategy. Those companies that depend on laboratory information can wait no longer to begin a large-scale commitment to LIMS because their competitors who have the commitment will have the advantage. We have stated that the justification of a LIMS should not be based on economic measures, but we should really use the phrase "short-term economics." In the long term, failure to commit to LIMS could have harsh economic effects. LIMS provides the means to automate information management. Those companies that depend on laboratory information, and are without a strategy that includes automated information management in their future, will be at the mercy not only of regulatory agencies but also of their competitors. The most successful manufacturing companies are now and always will be those that can beat their competitors to market with new products. This is true from the manufacture of alphabet soup, to pharmaceuticals, to retail goods, to zinc oxide. The rising standards of quality worldwide will demand more and more laboratory information — which means more and more laboratory data. If we try to manage the increases of data and resulting information with the same methods that we have been using since the 1970s, we will soon be out of business.

Many organizations attempt to justify a LIMS installation by economic measures. By finding fractions of workers' time which might be saved here and there, they compose a story using a laboratory wide sum of effort savings. After the LIMS is purchased and installed, implementation then becomes a political process. Much time is spent in selling the system to lab analysts, lab managers, other management, and potential LIMS users. Using political processes to promote LIMS use is a very complicated and expensive undertaking. Over time, the value of the LIMS will become apparent to all lab members who come in contact with it. However, the implementation will appear too lengthy. If support by upper management is not apparent to the LIMS team, even they might lose enthusiasm. If this happens, the project is in trouble.

As stated above, the investment in a LIMS is the implementation of a strategy. This is the justification for a LIMS. A LIMS is a strategy to remain competitive in the future. Who is better prepared to deal with strategies than top management? Strategy implementation and culture change require a vision of "the big picture" and an appreciation of long term investment. Thus, top management should be the driving force behind the LIMS implementation. Top management should implement the strategy, using a leadership process. Of course, many of the details of implementation will have to be solved by political means, but if support for the LIMS is top-down rather than bottom-up, implementation time will be dramatically reduced. Top management should counsel lab managers that the use of LIMS is part of the future strategy. Staffing the LIMS team with the required resources is a highly visible statement of support.

Summary

Installation and operation of LIMS are not cheap because they don't come with an on button. There are potential pitfalls and drawbacks. Some of the typical benefits which are expected from a LIMS are elimination of log books and paperwork, elimination of manual calculations, audit trails for data and information, data archival, and data assimilation. The worth of these benefits may not be obvious to all lab members. An educational process designed to give all lab members the opportunity to learn the value of laboratory information should be developed.

The installation of a LIMS is probably conceived as a major adjustment to lab processes by all lab members, and in many cases it is. Any reluctance by a lab manager to proceed with a LIMS installation is easily understood. A job component of each LIMS team member must be the requirement to spend as much time as needed in the lab working side by side with the analysts. There is absolutely no room for misunderstanding of how the LIMS functions work or which function is best in a particular situation. For example, if an analyst needs to enter test results for multiple samples for the same test, it will probably be faster to enter them by test code rather than by sample. An analyst unfamiliar with the LIMS might not recognize this. But the LIMS team member would know immediately if the wrong functions were being used. This is an example of a common misunderstanding that could be quickly spotted just by spending a little time in the lab.

Many organizations attempt to justify a LIMS implementation by using economic measures. The proper justification for a LIMS is related to having a vision of the future for the company. A LIMS implementation is a strategy for the future, and it requires a culture change. Leadership by top management is the best method to achieve the necessary commitment to ensure a successful LIMS project.

Section Five

Future Systems

Chapter 16

The Future of LIMS

Currently, LIMS are applying computing technology in the laboratory environment. They are reshaping existing methods of operation by making them more efficient through faster turnaround times and more sample throughput per analyst. They routinely provide information management tools to lab analysts, managers, and sample submitters. They are providing data repositories and data integrity, and they are allowing users to streamline resource allocation through automation. The time will come, however, when LIMS will no longer be making existing methods better. LIMS will evolve to the point of defining new methods of operation — but this sort of change takes time. It can't happen overnight — it takes years. At least we can be confident that we're on the right track.

We consider the management of all information in and around laboratories to be a new application technology. This new technology, born in the early 1980s, grew slowly through the mid 1980s without great furor. In the near future, no laboratory will be able to exist without it. LIMS, of course, is the new technology, and it is currently changing from being new to being commonplace. LIMS is built upon other computer application technologies which have already undergone the transformation, such as database technology and robotics. Other new, developing application technologies will have a major impact on future LIMS products. Some of these are windowing, object oriented database technology, and other artificial intelligence components such as knowledge based systems and voice recognition.

Invisible LIMS

For the next few years, the biggest problem facing those who install and use a LIMS is user acceptance, as described in Chapter 11. No matter how good the LIMS are, there will be those who are unwilling to use them simply because they are new and unfamiliar. Some laboratory workers will continue to use manual, paper-ridden methods, until they retire.

It has been suggested that one way to help solve the acceptance problem is to make the LIMS "user seductive" rather than just "user friendly." The system should make people want to use it. Better yet, the ideal LIMS should be "user invisible" for some functions. Lab members would interact with LIMS and not even know it. To illustrate the invisible LIMS concept, we will use the LOGIN function as an example.

Current Sample LOGIN Process

Before we can suggest anything new concerning the LIMS LOGIN function and associated behaviors, procedures, etc., we must first take a detailed look at what might be in use today. The following process, shown as a flowchart in Figure 16-1, illustrates the process which might be followed by a lab technician preparing samples and logging them into a LIMS:

1. Using a computer terminal in the lab, the technician logs in on the LIMS host computer system and initiates LIMS.
2. The technician chooses the LIMS sample LOGIN function from the LIMS main menu.
3. The user ID, sample type, test limits type, charge number, and required tests are entered into the LIMS at the terminal by using a laser scanner to scan a preprinted sheet of barcode labels containing these frequently used entries.
4. The sample ID is entered into the LIMS at the terminal by scanning a preprinted barcode label produced earlier by the technician.
5. The sample is transferred to a vial or envelope.
6. Sample-ID label is placed on the vial or envelope.
7. If there are more samples, begin again at step 3 or 4.
8. If there are no more samples, log out of LIMS.
9. Take the vial(s) or envelope(s) to the lab where the test(s) will be performed.

If a testing laboratory logs in its own samples, the procedures associated with sample LOGIN will certainly be different. There are probably as many variations to this LOGIN procedure as there are laboratories creating and/or receiving samples. However, we can still use this procedure to illustrate improvements which would be possible in many situations.

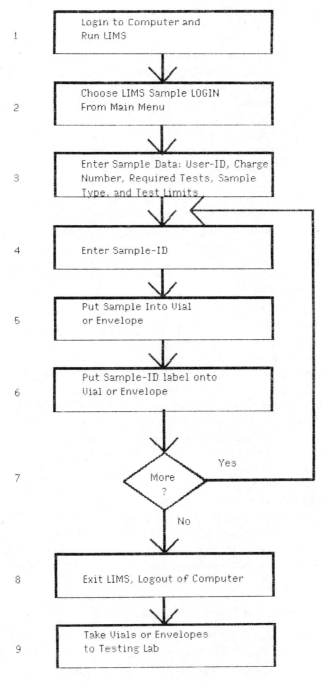

Figure 16-1. Sample preparation and LIMS LOGIN process.

Dedicated LIMS Terminal

The first thing we can do to make the technician's job more efficient is to eliminate step 1. This can be accomplished by placing a dedicated LIMS terminal in the lab. This terminal will always have the LIMS running and can always be looking for input. By using a touch screen, function keys, a mouse, or even a menu selection, the technician can begin a new LOGIN session at step 3 of the above process.

By using the dedicated terminal, we can also eliminate the entry of most or all of the items normally entered during sample LOGIN in step 3. The sample LOGIN function can be designed or tailored such that, under routine circumstances, it knows the user ID and can even provide logical defaults for the rest of the information. Thus, by pushing one or two keys on the terminal, the technician can quickly advance to step 4. Step 8 is also eliminated by using the dedicated terminal. The following, shown graphically in Figure 16-2, is the revised process using the dedicated LIMS terminal:

1. The technician chooses defaults by pushing one or two keys on the dedicated LIMS terminal.
2. The sample ID is entered into the LIMS at the terminal by scanning a preprinted barcode label produced earlier by the technician.
3. The sample is transferred to a vial or envelope.
4. The sample-ID label is placed on the vial or envelope.
5. If there are more samples, begin again at step 1 or 2.
6. If there are no more samples, take the vial(s) or envelope(s) to the lab where the test(s) will be performed.

The use of a terminal dedicated to a specific function is by no means a new idea. Point-of-sale terminals, airline reservation terminals, and other on-line transaction processing terminals are examples. Terminals are purchased and placed in labs for the sole purpose of using LIMS, but these can still be described as general purpose terminals. The concept of the dedicated terminal must be built into a LIMS. There are many other functions that could use a dedicated terminal, such as a quick-scan barcode reader, similar to grocery store checkout, for incoming samples.

Use of Barcodes and Their Limitations

There are two reasons for using barcode labels for the sample ID in the above processes. The first is to eliminate errors in sample ID processing. The technician can generate sample ID labels ahead of time in batch quantities. Then, by scanning the labels to enter the sample ID in LIMS

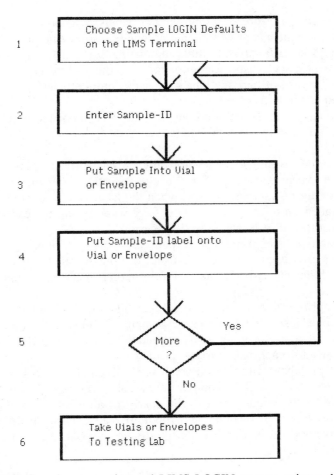

Figure 16-2. Sample preparation and LIMS LOGIN process using a dedicated LIMS terminal.

during sample LOGIN, transcription and other errors in sample IDs are almost totally eliminated. Elimination of sample ID errors is very important. If a sample is labeled incorrectly, test results may never be associated with the sample or extra time will be required at some point to figure out what went wrong. For example, the two sample numbers T-123456 and T123456 may appear functionally equal to the human mind, but to a computer they are not the same. If a sample was created and labeled T-123456 but was entered into the LIMS as T123456, later on, when test results are to be entered, the LIMS will not recognize the sample ID.

The second reason for using barcode labels is to provide a machine readable format which will enable automated processing later on when the samples are analyzed, thus eliminating some manual effort. And again, a primary reason for automation in the first place is to reduce errors. The use of barcode labels is clearly more efficient and desirable than paper methods.

Although barcodes are solutions to some very important problems, we are still faced with the following:

1. Barcode wand readers work only on flat surfaces. Laser readers are expensive (around $2000 each). A wand reader may be fine for use during sample LOGIN, when the label can be read before it is placed on a vial. But for later use, when trying to read the label on the vial, a laser reader is superior.
2. Barcode label printers are expensive relative to dot matrix printers. Dot matrix printers can be used, of course, but they won't print high density labels. They will print larger, medium- or low-density labels.
3. Preprinted labels can be small and high density, but it is hard to decide just what to preprint. Sample IDs must be unique. If you decide to preprint notebook page numbers as sample IDs, then how many for each page do you print?
4. Large labels won't fit on small vials. Even small labels are sometimes too big. This requires the use of envelopes on which to put the labels, which restricts the degree of automation later on. It is hard for even the nimblest robot to read a barcode label on an envelope, open the envelope, retrieve the vial, and place it in a vial holder.

Regardless of the problems associated with using barcode labels in the lab for sample IDs and other information, the cost and effort required are worth the investment. With the advances in robotics and automated sample processing, a LIMS without barcodes is like a bird without a song, a race car without an engine, or an Elvis without a guitar — it just isn't complete.

A Replacement for Peel and Stick Barcode Labels

The technological advances and achievements of barcodes have not yet peaked. Labels will get smaller, the number of characters packed per inch of label will increase, and the speed and reliability of readers will improve. Laser readers specifically designed to read small vials will soon be available. But the technology currently has an inherent drawback. In the laboratory, the labels must be peeled from their supporting medium and placed on the vial manually. There are currently machines which print, peel, and place barcode labels on boxes and larger items, and a similar machine to do the same with small lab containers is certainly feasible. So, until a machine is available to actually place the label on various sized vials, progress in automating lab processing will be restricted; however, we should begin thinking about future lab processes and what they will require.

Let's begin by considering methods of progressing beyond the peel and stick barcode label restriction. We have already mentioned one possible solution: use of a machine to place labels on vials automatically. Another solution is to use a machine-readable vial. This would allow us to encode information on the vial itself. It probably isn't feasible to require that sample vials be recycled. This would require expensive washing procedures. So, we still need inexpensive, disposable sample vials. Let's examine how a machine-readable vial might work:

1. Use vials made from magnetizable materials such as iron- or iron oxide-impregnated glass.
2. Use vials wrapped with a small piece of magnetizable tape.
3. Make a desktop machine which would wrap a small piece of magnetizable tape around a vial.
4. Create a "hot melt" solution or suspension of a magnetizable medium. Have a robot dip vials into the solution, either in batch mode off-line or just prior to using the vial.
5. Purchase sample vials from vendors already coated with the magnetizable substance.
6. (Don't forget optical media.) Use a sample vial containing a small optical disk, either on the bottom or the side.

In the case of magnetic media either on (or in) the vial itself or on an optical disk (or microdisk), we will need a machine containing read/write heads which would write (and read) the sample ID on the vial. In the case of automatically placed barcode labels, the machine would print the label and place it on the vial, and would probably have the ability to read what it had printed for verification. For either case, we will call our new machine a *vial-encoder machine*, or *VEM*.

Let's look at the sample LOGIN process using a VEM which automatically encodes the sample ID, any other needed information, on the vial itself. We don't have to be concerned with how it does it, only that the machine is connected to the computer and is driven by the LIMS. Figure 16-3 is a flowchart of the process, which is as follows:

1. The technician chooses defaults, including a new sample ID, by pushing one or two keys on the LIMS terminal.

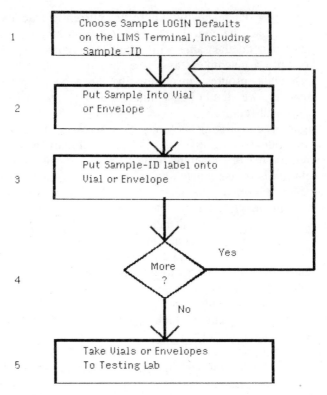

Figure 16-3. Sample preparation and LIMS LOGIN process using a dedicated LIMS terminal and a VEM.

2. Put the sample into a vial.
3. Put the vial into the VEM. The LIMS writes information to the vial.
4. If there are more samples, begin again at step 2.
5. If there are no more samples, take the vials to the lab where the tests will be performed.

Invisible LIMS and Other Functions

By using a terminal dedicated to LIMS applications, and assuming that we can design a LIMS to use it, we can effectively make the LIMS transparent to the user; thus, the LIMS becomes invisible. The technologies to build a VEM today can probably be found from several sources, and in fact, barcode technology is almost sufficient. Thus, the above exercise doesn't introduce any new technology, but only new application and methodology ideas.

The concept of the invisible LIMS can extend to nearly every LIMS function, from worklists to results reports. The important point to remember is that the LIMS must be part of the lab's natural way of doing business. If use of a LIMS can be blended into the lab's processes to the extent of being invisible, then we can be confident that the LIMS is in no way a hindrance and that it is making money for the lab. After a LIMS has been installed and personnel have used it long enough to climb the learning curve, if any lab member feels that the LIMS isn't helping, then the installation isn't finished. Invisibility won't be possible in every case or in every laboratory, but the LIMS must fit the lab.

New lab processes and procedures will always require learning and retraining, but new methods should never be implemented unless the end result is guaranteed to be more desirable than the old method. By blending a LIMS into existing processes and procedures, and making only minor changes where opportunities for improvement can be found, rejection can be minimized.

The Laboratory of the Future

The Software Revolution

Laboratory instruments and associated computer hardware will evolve over the coming years and take advantage of technology enhancements. Laboratory computer hardware, whether built into instruments or standing alone, will become more sophisticated and offer continuing advances in price/performance considerations. But regardless of how fast hardware advances dazzle our fancies, the next few years will see a software technology explosion the likes of which have never been known. We are only now seeing the beginning of the beginning of what will ultimately change the way all of us interact with computers. Hardware innovations have many strict physical limitations. But software, by contrast, has only one limitation: the imagination of its author.

As mentioned to in Chapter 2, the Apple Macintosh is a window on the future. The user interface, not hardware, will define the future of computing. This will have implications in every area of computing. For example, one significant area which will be affected is the operating system. There is currently a lot of controversy over the value and uses of the UNIX operating system. But in only a few years, the operating system won't matter. It won't matter if one uses an Open Software Foundation (OSF)-endorsed operating system or a vendor's proprietary operating system; in either case, the user interfaces will be the same. Users won't know what the operating system is, and they won't care. This view is shared by some persons in the computing industry who will have a major impact on product development over the next few years (58).

Laboratory computing is already able to take advantage of the software revolution. Results of "show-of-hands" surveys taken at the International LIMS Conferences (24,26) indicate that many laboratories, nearly half of those with representatives in attendance, already have LIMS in place and that a high percentage of the others plan to implement LIMS in the near future. Of the organizations with a LIMS already in place, those with commercial LIMS packages are in the best position to expect new software innovations sooner. Labs using in-house packages will be slower to obtain the new features. These labs will be forced to react to the software revolution in one of two ways: (1) by modifying existing programs to take advantage of new software innovations such as windowing, object-oriented databases, and knowledge based/intelligent systems, or (2) by scraping the in-house LIMS and acquiring a commercial package. Why will they be forced to accept one of these two options? To begin with, current LIMS vendors will be adopting new software features. If they don't, competition from new vendors, who will include every new feature possible, will put them out of business. For those labs with in-house written packages, pressure from lab scientists will force the LIMS support teams to implement solutions containing the new features. Scientists with Macintosh-like capability on their desks and at home will refuse to use an old technology LIMS.

Value Added Options

Some very innovative laboratory software is already available. In Chapter 7 we mentioned PE-Nelson's ACCESS*CHROM chromatography package. This software makes excellent use of windowing to work with chromatograms, and it also interfaces to ACCESS*LIMS. Although the chromatography package doesn't come with the LIMS, it can be considered an option. Options of this type will become more prevalent in the near future. While the LIMS vendors will move as quickly as they can to incorporate new software technology, they will also be offering more and more LIMS features, many of them as options. Modules for interfacing various instruments are another example of what we can expect to see as value-added features or options. The areas of software service, contract programming, and consulting will also become value-added "hot spots" in the LIMS arena as vendors realize their additional market potential.

Other modular offerings will very likely be the LIMS functions themselves. A site installing a LIMS would pick out the modules they want or possibly begin with a set of "core" LIMS functions offered as a starter package. All the modules would of course work together, and new ones could be added to provide additional capabilities. For example, a starter package might include sample LOGIN, worklists, results entry, results verification, and a standard results report. Optional modules might include archive, instrument interfacing, and additional reporting such as audit, backlog, and status reports.

We can look forward to the inclusion of molecular structure capability into LIMS. The results of many analytical tests, such as IR and NMR, are a combination of numeric, textural, and structure responses. LIMS users submitting samples for these tests routinely request structure conformations. They want to know, "Does the sample contain structure A?" The test result might be, "Yes, it does contain structure A, and also structure B."

A logical means of offering molecular structure capability with LIMS would be as an optional module. Not all LIMS users would need or want this capability. Production control and materials physical testing labs might not require the use of structures, whereas research labs in the pharmaceutical and chemical industries would certainly benefit from having it.

Automated Laboratory Instrumentation

In regulated environments, data acquisition systems to automatically acquire data and instrument management systems to control lab instruments will be required in years to come. LIMS have already begun to offer capability in this area, and future systems will showcase software and hardware technology breakthroughs in automated laboratory instrumentation. The development of new standards will provide the means for advancing instrument interfacing and data acquisition. Plug compatibility between instruments, computers, and LIMS will be achieved sooner or later. There have been radical changes in the seemingly aloof attitudes of laboratory products vendors over the past 10 years. These vendors are now encouraging standards and are investing the time and money to support standards organizations. In order to achieve meaningful standards sooner, rather than later, it is up to everyone working in the laboratory environment, both the vendors and their customers, to demand and support standards development.

There is a great need for radical changes and breakthroughs in automated laboratory instrumentation. In previous chapters, we have mentioned relatively new products for networking instruments, as well as new chromatography software which interfaces to a LIMS. These innovative new products may actually qualify as breakthroughs, and they are certainly indicators of things to come.

In the face of emerging laboratory instrumentation standards, the development of new proprietary methods does not hold much potential for vendors. Therefore, how can they justify the development expense? Within the next few years, the premier laboratory data products vendor(s) will be the one(s) implementing new methods which redefine laboratory automation. The laboratory computing market is ripe for a revolutionary redefinition of products, services, and features. Those innovators who are able to redefine the laboratory computing business by offering their customers orders-of-magnitude enhancements in features and, more importantly, service will succeed by leaping ahead of their competitors. There is currently plenty of room for leapers in this business.

How about an idea for a new feature to help with data acquisition? Many current lab instruments are capable of outputting data strings either to an attached PC or a printer. Other instruments are controlled by an external computer which collects data and creates a data file as part of the routine operation. Interfacing solutions being implemented today involve writing code to parse these captured files, extract the pertinent data, and store them in the LIMS database as results or test components. A very nice LIMS feature would be a function to indicate easily which data to extract from an instrument output data file. The function could display the data file on the terminal screen and allow the LIMS user to select and name the desired data fields by simply highlighting them, using a mouse. The LIMS would then know from which rows and columns to extract test components, peak names, raw data, etc.

Automated Laboratory Information Management

LIMS are the tools with which to build automated laboratory information management for today and tomorrow. LIMS will not remain a new technology for long. They will soon be commonplace and a part of every laboratory. The significant worldwide interest in LIMS has begun to generate new LIMS products, new LIMS features, and even new companies dealing with LIMS. The most significant advances in laboratory information management in the immediate future will be in the acceptance of LIMS by all laboratory members. Until now, LIMS projects have always begun with a cost/benefit justification study. In the near future, traditional businesses which have relied on laboratory support will be changing. The successes of the chemical and pharmaceutical industries will soon (if not already) depend on information management. As a result, the operation of a laboratory without a LIMS in place will be questioned. Information management is now the name of the game. For some industries, the management of laboratory information will make the difference between success and failure.

Even with the progress which LIMS has enabled for laboratory information management, a redefinition of information management is still needed. Those innovative lab data products and LIMS vendors which, over the next few years, reinvent methods of data management, customer information management, and applications of LIMS supervisory functions will thrive. Those which don't will either die or will find themselves scrambling for a share of the market as they try to catch up. The potential to double and redouble the size of the LIMS market exists. The rate of delivery of innovative new products and services will drive the market expansion faster than any other factor.

Integration

Computing in the laboratory of the future will be integrated. Application programs will be integrated with LIMS and other application programs. Applications in one laboratory will be integrated with applications in others. Lab instruments will be integrated into computer networks. Integration and networking are currently strategic directions for computer and lab data products vendors. As we plan for future LIMS, integration of every component possible must be considered.

LIMS itself is a collection of integrated tools, with the database being the common factor of integration. As we implement solutions to data handling and information management problems by customizing or adding new LIMS functions, we must always look for opportunities to integrate these solutions. For example, if LIMS users need to evaluate test results using statistical processes, the LIMS must be integrated with an external software system which provides the necessary capability. To the LIMS user, the system must function as a single tool, not as a collection of independent solutions. Integration to the highest degree possible, at the expense of time and effort, is an investment which cannot be put off or eliminated. If it is necessary to justify the effort required to integrate a particular data- or information management-related solution into a LIMS, a return in the range of 200–400% a year or more can be anticipated.

Computer Systems Validation

The validation of computer systems is already required in some environments. Over the next decade, more and more laboratories will be implementing SOPs and validation protocols for their computer systems. Logically, a LIMS should contain functions and features to assist its users in applying these validation processes. A major aspect of computer system validation is *ongoing system evaluation*. This task can be simplified by having the LIMS schedule standard samples at regular, predefined intervals and automatically compare the results with previous data to guarantee that the operation is continuing as expected. Database integrity and security can be periodically tested by submitting complex searches to test data relations and access privileges.

The users of commercial LIMS are currently relying on vendors to provide thorough, well-tested solutions with all the data integrity and security needed to meet even the strictest validation protocol. But currently, the user has the sole responsibility for implementing a validation protocol and guaranteeing compliance with it. This responsibility must be shared by the LIMS vendors in future laboratory environments. Although LIMS are computer applications, they are still merely tools for lab personnel. These individuals cannot be responsible for testing and validating commercial LIMS. They should only be responsible for using a LIMS product which has been certified as compliant with a LIMS performance standard. Thus, commercial products must be designed and marketed as being compliant with the standard. The standard will emerge in the 1990s.

LIMS: The Next Generations

We are currently well into the use of the second generation of LIMS. The third generation will be available by 1991. About the fourth generation, we can only guess. The characteristics of these generations are as follows:

First-Generation LIMS

- Begin — early 1970s with in-house written systems
- End — early 1980s
- First commercial LIMS as we know them today — around 1980
- Widespread use of instrument interfacing — late 1970s

Second-Generation LIMS

- Begin — early 1980s
- End — around 1990
- Designed to interface instruments
- Use of multiuser, general-purpose, database products not specifically designed for the LIMS, such as third-party database
- First use of networking — around 1987
- First use of robotics — around 1986
- Beginning of integration of LIMS and external applications

Third-Generation LIMS

- Begin — around 1990
- End — around 1993?
- Extensive use of networking
- Use of windows and Macintosh-type user interface
- Easier instrument interfacing
- Begin use of knowledge-based, intelligent functions
- Emphasis on automating information management features such as instrument management and other supervisory function
- Extensive integration of LIMS and external applications

Fourth-Generation LIMS

- Begin — around 1993?
- Simple instrument interfacing
- Use of voice recognition
- Extensive use of knowledge-based, intelligent functions
- Self-validating
- Intelligent integration of LIMS and external applications

We stated above that there is room for innovative, new LIMS functions to redefine laboratory data processing. Hopefully, we will begin seeing enhancements of this magnitude by the beginning of the fourth generation. In fact, these significant enhancements may actually define the beginning of the fourth generation. Some of them will assuredly take the form of intelligent systems such as knowledge-based and voice recognition systems. Others will make LIMS implementation and support much easier with simplified instrument interfacing.

The main point to remember when trying to envision future LIMS products, applications, and features is that LIMS will be commonplace in the future. There will be no justification necessary for LIMS as we know them today. Automating instrumentation and information management using LIMS will be the standard. For example, instruments will be sold with software modules to interface them to LIMS using standards developed by standards organizations such as ASTM. But this isn't to say that other new computer products and processes won't come along that will require justification.

Other Products and Features

Within 10 years, it is certain that new sets of laboratory data products will emerge. Some of them will be spurred by developments in instrumentation, some by developments in software, and some by developments in computer hardware. LIMS will no longer be a new application technology but will likely be a built-in part of these new data products. Robotics will advance to the point where LIMS/robot interface modules will be offered by both LIMS and robot vendors — which are the same in some cases. We must assume that instrumentation will continue to be augmented with faster computer hardware and innovative new software to enable more data to be collected and processed.

Encompassing molecular structure capability into LIMS might initially be accomplished by building a LIMS solution which integrates multiple software products from multiple sources — such as a LIMS from a LIMS vendor and an in-house written graphics package. The hardware to support the use of structures must be considered. Currently, effective graphics processing is relatively expensive. Structures can be displayed on graphics terminals costing less than $2000, but a fast, easy to use graphics editor would be required for use with the LIMS in order to draw structures. PCs and low end workstations can provide this graphics editing function, but they cost from $4000 to $20,000. In order for use of molecular structures to become routine and widespread within laboratories, the cost of a workstation must be less than $2000. In order for the cost to be less than $2000, the workstation would probably be diskless, thus requiring it to be networked to a minicomputer. Graphics data, such as structures, have a high storage requirement. The network will provide access to this large storage requirement. Optical storage technology, because of its high-volume data capacity, will be a welcome addition to the LIMS computing environment for storage and archival requirements.

Software innovations will enhance future LIMS. Distributed databases will take advantage of high-speed networked workstations to offer shared data availability without a central CPU. Object oriented database technology will use workstation graphics to speed use of molecular structures. Knowledge based system enhancements to data retrieval, instrument interfacing, user set up, and report generation will be applied to LIMS in the near future by user customization, and hopefully in the commercial packages as well.

Summary

In the end, when all is said and done, LIMS is big business. Whether we choose to write our own LIMS or purchase and customize/tailor a commercial package, the LIMS business will affect laboratory operations for a long time to come. The opportunity represented by the LIMS business is enormous. Total revenue from LIMS sales will increase every year for many years to come as LIMS use becomes the standard. The combination of Perkin Elmer and Nelson Systems is an example of a business endeavor to gain a strategic position in the lab data products and LIMS markets. We will see more mergers, cooperative projects and products, and more positioning between the large forces in the lab data products business. Forging a successful new startup business in this area will be extremely difficult, as it always has been. Startups don't last long. If they're not successful, they merely close shop. If they are successful, they are likely to be bought out.

Some existing products, even some of the ones used in previous chapters to highlight features, will become obsolete and will cease to be offered. New product offerings will take their place. Some existing products will last for many years. The survivors will be the ones that incorporate new features and technologies as rapidly as possible, and whose vendors figure out how to provide customer service beyond our wildest dreams.

The software revolution will sweep through the laboratories in the next 10 years. The user interface, as we know it at the start of the 1990s, will be totally replaced. This interface has already become the primary focus for software development activities.

The LIMS vendors will do what is necessary to sell their products. But this is good for companies that depend on laboratory information. These companies have always paid a premium for laboratory products, from glassware to instruments, and lab data products are no exception. Expectations of high quality and high standards have accompanied the high prices. The best we, the end users, can hope for is that the LIMS business remains highly competitive.

References

1. Bayer, S., and Iorns, T. 1987. LIMS — Lab Data Management: Are They The Same? *Sci. Comput. Automat.* 4(1):23.
2. Martin, G.E. 1986. A LIMS with a Strategic Focus. *Am. Lab.* 18(2):98.
3. Mahaffey, R.R. 1987. Applying LIMS in the Analytical Laboratory. *Am. Lab.* 19(9):82.
4. Scott, F.I., Jr. 1987. Data Management Functions in LIMS. *Am. Lab.* 19(11):50.
5. Bayer, S., and Iorns, T. 1987. Lab Data Management Systems and Laboratory Information Management Systems Buyer's Guide. *Sci. Comput. Automat.* 4(1):36.
6. Ackoff, R.L. 1981. *Creating the Corporate Future.* New York: John Wiley & Sons.
7. Drucker, P.F. 1968. *The Age of Discontinuity.* New York: Harper & Row.
8. Toffler, A. 1971. *Future Shock.* New York: Bantam Books.
9. Schon, D.A. 1971. *Beyond the Stable State.* New York: Random House.
10. Food and Drug Administration. 1983. *Guide to Inspection of Computerized Systems in Drug Processing.* U.S. Dept. of Health and Human Services: Washington, D.C.
11. Food and Drug Administration. 1976. Current GMP in the Manufacture, Processing, Packing, or Holding of Large-Volume Parenterals. *Fed. Register.* 41(6):22202.
12. Chapman, K.G., Harris, J.R., Bluhm, A.R., and Errico, J.J. 1989. Source Code Availability and Vendor-User Relationships. *Pharm. Tech.* 11(12).
13. Masters, G., and Figarole, P. 1986. Validation Principles for Computer Systems — FDA's Perspective. *Pharm. Tech.* 10(11):44.
14. Clark, A.S. 1988. Computer Systems Validation: An Investigator's View. *Pharm. Tech.* 12(1):60.
15. Motise, P.J. 1984. What to Expect When FDA Audits Computer-Controlled Processes. *Pharm. Manuf.* ( ):33.
16. Motise, P.J. 1984. Validation of Computerized Systems in the Control of Drug Processes: An FDA Perspective. Pharm. Tech. 8(3):40.
17. Pharmaceutical Manufacturers Association, Computer Systems Validation Committee. 1986. Validation Concepts for Computer Systems Used in the Manufacture of Drug Products. *Pharm. Tech.* 10(5):24.
18. Food and Drug Administration. 1987. *Technical Reference on Software Development Activities.* U.S. Dept. of Health and Human Services: Washington, D.C.

19. Kuzel, N.R. 1985. Fundamentals of Computer System Validation and Documentation in the Pharmaceutical Industry. *Pharm. Tech.* 9(9):60.
20. Martin, J. 1984. *An Information Systems Manifesto*. Englewood Cliffs, N.J.: Prentice-Hall.
21. Agalloco, J. 1987. Validation of Existing Computer Systems. *Pharm. Tech.* 11(1):38.
22. Hewlett-Packard Company. 1985. LABSAM Audit Trail System Reference Manual. Palo Alto, Calif. pp. 4-5.
23. Food and Drug Administration. 1985. Computerized Drug Processing: Source Code for Process Control Application Programs. *Compliance Policy Guide 7132a.15*. U.S. Dept. of Health and Human Services: Washington, D.C.
24. First International LIMS Meeting. June 1987. Pittsburgh.
25. Murkitt, G.S. 1987. The LIMS Organization. In *Laboratory Information Management Systems, Concepts, Integration, Implementation*, ed. McDowall, R.D. Wilmslow, England: Sigma Press, pp 57-66.
26. Second International LIMS Meeting. June 1988. Pittsburgh.
27. Axiom Systems, Inc. 1988. *VM LIMS Reference Manual Administrative Functions*. East Meadow, N.Y. p 1-CT.
28. Beckman Instruments, Inc. *Laboratory Information Management and Data Acquisition System*. Waldwick, N.J. p 25-27.
29. PE-Nelson Systems, Inc. 1988. *System Specifications for ACCESS*LIMS*. Cupertino, Calif. p 42.
30. Ryan, J.F. 1988. Quality Assurance Applications for Laboratory Information Management Systems. Presented at the 102nd Association of Official Analytical Chemists (AOAC) Meeting. Palm Beach, Florida. August 30.
31. Megargle, R. 1988. Pitfalls and Possibilities During the Acquisition of a LIMS. Presented at the 102nd Association of Official Analytical Chemists (AOAC) Meeting. Palm Beach, Florida. August 31.
32. Chesapeake Software, Inc. Consultants in the Computer Sciences. Brandywood Plaza. Suite 221. 2500 Grubb Road. Wilmington, Del. 19810.
33. St. Clair, D. 1984. Network and Communications. In *Computers in the Laboratory*, ed. Liscouski, J.G. Washington, D.C.:American Chemical Society. pp. 37-44.
34. Megargle, R., quoted by Cannon, D.R. 1987. To Get Ready for LIMS: Look Before You Leap. *Indust. Chemist.* 8(4):28.
35. Mansfield, P., quoted by Cannon, D.R. 1987. To Get Ready for LIMS: Look Before You Leap, *Indust. Chemist* 8(4):28.
36. Mansfield, P., Berthrong, P., Kipiniak, W., Wheaton, S., Voelkner, R., and Karlan, D. 1986. A Third-Generation Chromatography Automation System. *Am. Lab.* 18(2):107.
37. Liscouski, J.G. 1988. Issues and Directions in Laboratory Automation *Anal. Chem.* 60:95A.
38. Cooper, E.L., and Turkel, E.J. 1988. Performance of a Paperless Laboratory. *Am. Lab.* 20(3):42.
39. Davis, A., Belton, G., and Matthews, D. 1988. Interfacing Laboratory Instruments to a LIMS Computer System. *Am. Lab.* 20(9):34.
40. Janney, R., Davis, C., Brencovich, E., and Gilmore, T. 1988. Instrument Data Acquisition. *Am. Lab.* 20(3):34.

41. Berthrong, P.G., and Mansfield, P.B. 1986. Automation Systems for Small Laboratories: Part Two, Nonchromatographic Data and LIMS Functions. *Am. Lab.* 18(5):82

42. Santori, M., and Vento, T. 1988. Words, Spreadsheets, and Pictures: Three Data Acquisition Software Methods for Laboratory Automation. *Am. Lab.* 20(9):78.

43. Levy, B., and Herrick, S. 1988. LIMS in the Corporate Environment. Part 1: Competence in the Laboratory. *Am. Lab.* 20(9):86.

44. Hampshire, A.1987. Databases. In *Laboratory Information Management Systems, Concepts, Integration, Implementation,* ed. McDowall, R.D. Wilmslow, England: Sigma Press, pp. 102-127.

45. PE-Nelson Systems, Inc. 1988. *System Specifications for ACCESS*LIMS.* Cupertino, Calif.

46. Digital Equipment Corporation. 1987. *VAX LIMS/SM Users Guide.* Maynard, Mass.

47. Varian Associates. 1986. *Varian Laboratory Data Management User's Manual.* Varian LIMS/DM Version 1.7.1. Walnut Creek, Calif.

48. Crisp S.B., and Mollner J. 1987. LABSAM. In *Laboratory Information Management Systems, Concepts, Integration, Implementation,* ed. McDowall, R.D. Wilmslow England: Sigma Press. pp. 102-127.

49. Head, M., and Smith, K. 1988. A Network Data Acquisition System. *Am. Lab.* 20(8):62.

50. PE-Nelson Systems, Inc. *ACCESS*CHROM The Chromatography Data System For VAX Computers.* Cupertino, Calif.

51. Welch, V.F. 1988. *LIMS Overview.* LIMS Video Training. Eastman Chemicals Division, Eastman Kodak Company. Kingsport, Tenn.

52. Digital Equipment Corporation. 1987. *VAX LIMS/SM Planning Workbook.* Maynard, Mass.

53. Reynolds, J. 1988. MIS Managers Must See Themselves Honestly. *Computerworld.*

54. Digital Equipment Corporation. 1987. *VAX LIMS/SM Manager's Guide.* Maynard, Mass.

55. Branning, R.C. 1987. Computer Systems Validation — How to Get Started. *Pharm. Eng.* 7(3):11.

56. Howard, M. 1988. Computer Integrated Manufacturing. Presented at the Eastman Chemicals Division, Eastman Kodak Company. November, 15.

57. Beckman Instruments Inc. 1987. CALS Lab Manager — An Advanced Laboratory Information Management System with a History of Success. *Bulletin 7991.* Waldwick, N.J. p 9.

58. Olsen, K. 1988. Integrating the Enterprise. Presented at Gartner Group Conference. Washington D.C., December 5.

59. *Webster's New World Dictionary, Second College Edition.* 1970. New York:The World Publishing Company.

60. Cash, J., McFarlan, W., and McKenney, J. 1988. *Corporate Information Systems Management.* Homewood, Ill.:IRWIN

Appendixes

Appendix A-1[1]

How LIMS/DM Tracks Samples and Tests

Among different laboratories, there exists a wide variety of testing facilities with many potential configurations of laboratory workstations, instruments, analysts, and testing methods. The core function, however, of any laboratory is basically the same, to move samples from their log-in to the final reporting and archiving of test results through the laboratory. LIMS/DM divides this fundamental workflow into a series of definite changes in sample and test statuses, or states, which are analogous to the familiar and fundamental sequence of actions performed in all laboratories.

These sample and test states allow you to track the progress of sample and test processing. The Sample Directory or Sample Status functions can be used in order to display the statuses of selected samples and tests in the database. Also, the LIMS/DM Select function can be used to display the statuses of tests which are not yet complete.

The Sample States

The following paragraphs describe the sample states that are assigned as samples flow through the LIMS/DM system. Figure A-1 presents a flowchart of the sample states used by LIMS/DM. When you are using LIMS/DM, the current statuses of the samples and tests can be checked by using the Sample Status and Sample Directory functions.

Sample "IN-LAB" (IL)

A sample status of In-Lab (IL) is given to a sample that has been logged into LIMS/DM (on the Login Sample screen), but does not have any tests that are currently assigned to a Worklist. As soon as any of the tests requested for the sample are placed on a Worklist, the sample status will change to In-Test (IT). Any tests requested for a sample that have been put on Hold (Test status set to Hold (HO) on the Login Hold screen) are not considered to be assigned to a Worklist.

[1] Reprinted with permission: Varian Associates. 1986. How Varian LIMS/DM Tracts Samples and Tests. *Varian Laboratory Data Management User's Manual*. Varian LIMS/DM Version 1.7.1 pages 4-8 through 4-14.

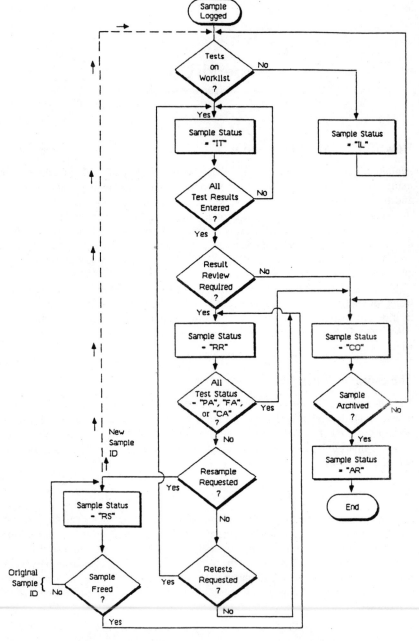

Figure A-1. LIMS/DM Sample State Flowchart (Varian Associates. 1986. *Varian Laboratory Data Management User's Manual*. Varian LIMS/DM. Version 1.7.1. Walnut Creek, Calif. p. 4-9)

Sample "IN-TEST" (IT)

While any of the tests requested for a sample are listed on a Worklist, the sample state is In-Test (IT). The sample state will remain In-Test until the results for all its requested tests have been entered into or transmitted to LIMS/DM. A sample in the In-Test (IT) test state cannot be canceled.

Sample "REVIEW REQUIRED" (RR)

The Review Required (RR) sample state indicates that the LIMS/DM Review function should be used to examine, and pass or fail, the results of one or more of the completed tests assigned to the sample. A sample will enter the Review Required (RR) state when the results for all of the sample's non-canceled tests have been entered into or transmitted to LIMS/DM, and the status of one or more of the tests is Review Required (RR). Some LIMS/DM samples may never enter the Review Required state. For example, if none of the tests assigned to a sample uses a Method–Section which requires review, the sample will go directly from In-Test to Completed as soon as all non-canceled tests assigned to the sample have been completed.

Sample "RESAMPLE" (RS)

A sample will enter the Resample (RS) state if there is a request for resampling on a Review screen. Requesting a resample will automatically log in a new sample with the same test and Worklist assignments as the original sample. The original sample will stay in the Resample (RS) state until the sample is released ("Freed") on the Review screen.

Sample "COMPLETED" (CO)

A sample enters the Completed (CO) sample state when the test state of all tests assigned to the sample are Passed (PA), Failed (FA), Analyzed (AN), or Canceled (CA). Tests are Passed (PA) or Failed (FA) on a Review screen and are Canceled (CA) on the Login Cancel screen. Tests performed using a Method–Section which does not require review, become Analyzed (AN) when the results for all components of the test are entered or transmitted to LIMS/DM.

Sample "ARCHIVED" (AR)

If the LIMS/DM Database Archive function has been used to store a sample's test results onto an external storage device (tape or disk), the sample state becomes Archived (AR). A record of the archived sample remains in the LIMS/DM database, but the results of the tests that were assigned to the archived sample are moved to a disk or tape storage device and are not available unless the Utility Retrieve function is used to restore the sample's test results to the LIMS/DM database.

Sample "HOLD" (HO)

A sample can be placed in the Hold (HO) state on the Login Hold screen in order to temporarily indicate that further work should not be performed on the sample. When a sample is placed on Hold, all tests assigned to the sample, with the exception of Pending (PE) and In-Tests tests, will be given a test status of Hold (HO). Pending (PE) and In-Test (IT) tests will not be put on Hold until the tests leave these states. The Hold sample state will be maintained until the Login Release function is used to release the sample. Samples which have a sample status of Archived, Canceled, or Resample may not be put on Hold.

Sample "CANCELED" (CA)

A sample that has been canceled on the Login Cancel screen is given a sample status of Canceled (CA). All tests assigned to a canceled sample, with the exception of Pending (PE) and In-Test (IT) tests, are immediately given a test status of Canceled (CA). Pending (PE) and In-Test (IT) tests are canceled (CA) as soon as they leave these states. Canceling a sample permanently prevents LIMS/DM system actions, with the exception of sample archiving, from being performed upon the sample or its tests.

The Test States

Tests which have been assigned to samples logged into LIMS/DM go through a series of distinctive test states similar to the sample states just described. These test states indicate the current stage of test processing. The states of tests assigned to samples logged into LIMS/DM may be displayed by using the Sample Directory function or the Status function. Both of these functions display the sample and test states of selected samples.

The following paragraphs define the test states used in LIMS/DM.

Test "IN-LAB" (IL)

If a test has been requested for a sample, but the test is not assigned to a Worklist, the state is In-Lab. After the test has been assigned to a Worklist, its state will become Selected (SE).

Test "SELECTED" (SE)

When a test requested for a sample has been assigned to a Worklist, but not yet "activated" for analysis on a LIMS/DM Select screen, the state of the test is Selected (SE).

Test "PENDING" (PE)

When a test on a Worklist is ready for an actual analysis, you can "activate" the test on a LIMS/DM Select screen. When a test is activated, its test state changes from Selected (SE) to Pending (PE) and LIMS/DM will accept the results of the test.

Test "IN-TEST" (IT)

The In-Test (IT) test state is reserved for tests which receive their results from an analytical instrument or data station. A Pending (PE) test on a Worklist will become In-Test (IT) when LIMS/DM receives the test results from the instrument or data station and stores them in its database. How long a test stays in the In-Test state depends upon whether or not the Worklist to which the test is assigned has a Worklist Completion Procedure:

If the Worklist has a Worklist Completion Procedure, the test will remain In-Test (IT) until results for all Pending (PE) tests on the Worklist have been received and the Worklist Completion Procedure has executed. Following the execution of the Worklist Completion Procedure, the In-Test (IT) tests will become either Review Required(RR) or Analyzed (AN), depending upon whether or not the assigned Method–Sections have been configured as Review Required.

If the Worklist does not have a Worklist Completion Procedure, the test will briefly remain In-Test (IT), and will then be given a status of Review Required(RR) or Analyzed (AN), depending upon whether or not the assigned Method–Section has been configured as Review Required.

For information on the Worklist Completion Procedures and Method – Section configuration, refer to the LIMS/DM Managers Manual. For information on the use of the LIMS/DM Instrument function, see Chapter 8 of this manual.

Test "Analyzed" (AN)

If the Method–Section used for a test has been configured as not requiring review, the test's state will become Analyzed (AN) when the results for all components of the test have been entered into or transmitted to LIMS/DM.

Test "REVIEW REQUIRED" (RR)

If the Method–Section used for a test has been configured as requiring review, the test's state will become Review Required (RR) when the results for all components of a test have been entered into or transmitted to the system. The Review Required test state will be maintained until some action (Pass, Fail, Retest, or Resample) is taken on a Review screen.

Test "PASSED" (PA)

When the results of a test in the Review Required (RR) test state are passed on a Review screen, the state of the test will become Passed (PA).

Test "FAILED" (FA)

When the results of a test in the Review Required (RR) test state of failed (FA) on a Review screen, the state of the test becomes Failed (FA).

Test "RETEST" (RT)

When the results of a test in the Review Required (RR) test state are questionable, and a retest is requested on a Review screen, the state of the test will become Retest (RT). The test will stay in the Retest state until the test is released ("freed"). It can then be Passed, Failed, Canceled, put on Hold, or Resampled.

Test "RESAMPLE" (RS)

If a resample is requested on a Review screen, the statuses of all tests assigned to the sample will become Resample (RS). Also, a new sample is automatically logged in and assigned the same tests as the sample for which the resample was requested. The state of all tests assigned to the original sample will remain RS until the sample is released ("freed") on the Review screen. When the sample is released ("freed"), all tests will revert to their previous states. See Chapter 9 for a further description of the use of the Review function.

Test "HOLD" (HO)

If the Login Hold screen is used to hold a test, its test state will become Hold (HO). A test state of Hold is also assigned to the tests of a sample put on Hold (Sample State set to Hold on the Login Hold screen). Tests cannot be put on Hold if the sample has a state of Archived, Canceled, or Resample. A Pending or In-Test test will not be given a status of Hold until the test leaves the Pending or In-Test state.

Test "CANCELED" (CA)

If a test is canceled on the Login Cancel Screen, its test state becomes Canceled (CA). A test also has a status of Canceled if the sample to which the test was assigned has a sample status of Canceled. Tests with statuses of Pending or In-Test are not actually given a status of Canceled until the tests leave the Pending or In-Test states.

Appendix A-2

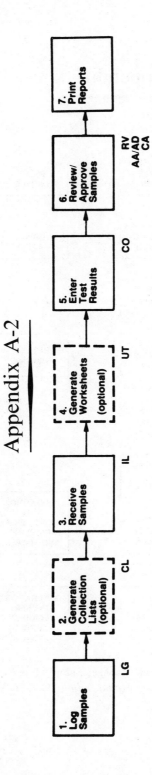

Figure A-2. DEC LIMS/SM Sample Processing Flow (Digital Equipment Corp. 1987. *VAX LIMS/SM Planning Workbook*. Maynard, Mass. p. 1-6)

Appendix A-3

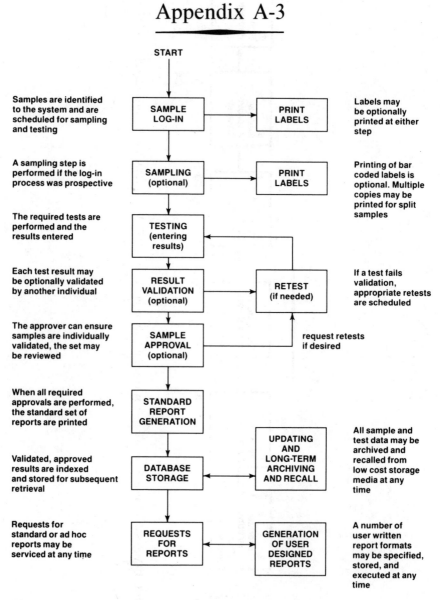

START

Samples are identified to the system and are scheduled for sampling and testing	**SAMPLE LOG-IN** → **PRINT LABELS**	Labels may be optionally printed at either step
A sampling step is performed if the log-in process was prospective	**SAMPLING (optional)** → **PRINT LABELS**	Printing of bar coded labels is optional. Multiple copies may be printed for split samples
The required tests are performed and the results entered	**TESTING (entering results)**	
Each test result may be optionally validated by another individual	**RESULT VALIDATION (optional)** → **RETEST (if needed)**	If a test fails validation, appropriate retests are scheduled
The approver can ensure samples are individually validated, the set may be reviewed	**SAMPLE APPROVAL (optional)**	request retests if desired
When all required approvals are performed, the standard set of reports are printed	**STANDARD REPORT GENERATION**	
Validated, approved results are indexed and stored for subsequent retrieval	**DATABASE STORAGE** ↔ **UPDATING AND LONG-TERM ARCHIVING AND RECALL**	All sample and test data may be archived and recalled from low cost storage media at any time
Requests for standard or ad hoc reports may be serviced at any time	**REQUESTS FOR REPORTS** ↔ **GENERATION OF USER DESIGNED REPORTS**	A number of user written report formats may be specified, stored, and executed at any time

Figure A-3. Beckman CALS Lab Manager Sample Processing Flow (Beckman Instruments, Inc.1987. *CALS Lab Manager Bulletin 7991*. Waldwick, N.J. p. 5)

238

Appendix A-4

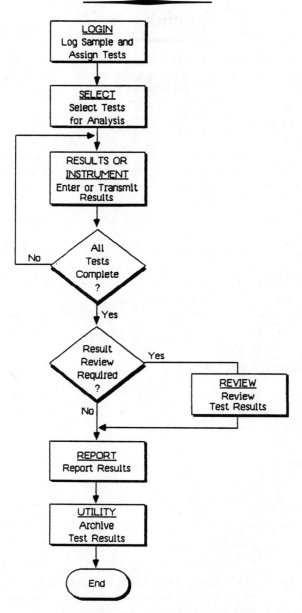

Figure A-4. Varian LIMS/DM Sample Processing Flow (Varian Associates. 1986. *Varian Laboratory Data Management User's Manual.* Varian LIMS/DM Version 1.7.1. Walnut Creek. p 4-7)

Appendix A-5

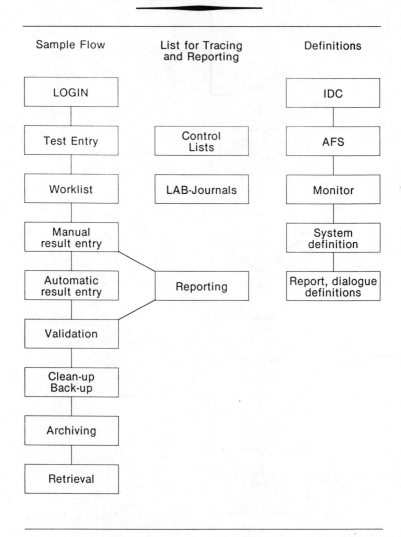

Figure A-5. HP LABSAM System Overview (Crisp, S.B, and Mollner, J. 1987. LABSAM. In *Laboratory Information Management Systems*, ed. R.D. Mc-Dowall., Wilmslow, England:Sigma Press, p. 266)

Appendix B

Glossary

Algorithm. Equation or combination of logic and equations designed to provide a solution to a particular problem or set of problems.

Aliquot. A portion of a sample. Some LIMS provide the capability of reporting test results for aliquots.

Analysis. A "test" performed upon a sample to determine its composition or other characterizing traits.

Analyst. Laboratory member usually directly involved with sample analysis.

Approval. Examination and acceptance of sample test results.

Archive. Store data off-line. The data is usually removed from the active database and placed onto magnetic tape or removable disks.

Auditing. Assuring the integrity of data by maintaining a revision history.

Audit Trail. A revision history of sample test results and associated data maintained such that any modifications are accompanied by who, when, and why they were made.

Backlog. Work remaining to be done, or samples remaining to be processed.

Barcode Label. A label usually produced on peel-and-stick paper. The label is composed of a machine readable code and usually contains sample-ID in LIMS related processing.

Barcode Reader. A machine which reads barcode labels.

Batch. A group of items considered as one unit. In LIMS, batch processing indicates the processing of several samples as a unit at the same time.

CODASYL. Acronym for Conference On Data Systems Languages. It is used to describe an industry-wide specification for database design.

Collection List. List of samples ready to be collected and distributed to a testing laboratory or laboratories.

Collector. Individual collecting samples for distribution to a testing laboratory or laboratories.

Component. A physical or analytical test may determine several data items. A single item is considered a component.

Cursor. The blinking, or highlighted, "current position" indicator of a video computer terminal.

Customizing. Extensive modification of a computer program or computer system, such as a LIMS.

Data. Any information related to samples, instruments, customers, analysts, labs, or other LIMS related objects.

Data Entry. The entry of data into a computer, or LIMS, by either manual (keyboard) or automated methods.

Data Management System. Processes, which make use of computer programs to collect, store, and make use of laboratory data.

Database. A collection of logically related information maintained by a set of computer programs designed for efficient storage and retrieval.

Default. Information which is automatically provided, which will be accepted unless overridden.

Device. Laboratory instrument.

Field. Designated space on a video terminal screen for entry of a particular data item.

File. Computer system storage location, usually a disk file.

GLP. Good Laboratory Practices. Initially designed by the FDA to define desirable laboratory procedures in drug testing laboratories.

GMP. Good Manufacturing Practices. Initially designed by the FDA to define desirable procedures in drug manufacturing and related quality assurance.

Instrument. Device for measuring properties of a physical sample.

Instrument Management System. Processes which make use of computer programs to properly maintain laboratory instruments. Maintenance schedules and standard sample scheduling with statistical analysis are components of instrument management.

Limit. Maximum or minimum deviation from a statistically expected result.

LIMS Function. An integral part of a LIMS, such as sample LOGIN and RE-SULTS ENTRY.

Location. A particular area which generates samples. The location is important when collection lists are used.

Manual Data Entry. Keyboard entry of data into a LIMS.

Menu. List of items or functions from which to choose.

Method. Physical or analytical testing procedure.

Privilege. The right to use a particular LIMS function or feature.

Prompt. A message or indication that input is required.

Protocol. A procedure or set of specifications which describe a desired output or product.

Query. A question (or set of questions) either from a computer system to a user, or from a user to a computer system. A database query is a database search done to answer a certain question (or set of questions).

Raw Data. The first set of results from a physical or analytical test, before any data reductions or calculations are performed.

Record. A single, complete, entry in a database.

Relational Database. Database consisting of a set of tables (relations) which are related to each other according to field values.

Report. Compilation of results for a sample or samples. Result reports are usually distributed to the sample submitter by the testing lab.

Result. Usually the final outcome of a physical or analytical test. Raw data can sometimes be referred to as results.

Retest.   A repeat of a test for some reason – either requested by the analyst, the result reviewer, or by the sample submitter.

Retrieve.   Access of sample information or other data which has been archived.

Review.   To examine test results in order to verify their correctness. If correct, they would be released to the sample submitter. If not correct, a retest might be scheduled.

Revision History.   After a test result has been entered into the LIMS database, any revision to that result must be accompanied by who made the revision, when it was made, and why. This record is the revision history.

Route.   The path to be followed by a sample collector, indicating locations for sample pick up and delivery.

Run Number.   When a sample is submitted more than once, for the same test, the run number is used to keep track of the multiple results. The run number is 1 for the first test, 2 for the second, etc.

Sample.   A physical specimen of something, which is to be analyzed by some physical or analytical test.

Sample ID.   Unique identifier which is assigned to a sample, usually by the sample creator.

Sample Management System.   Processes which make use of computer programs to help maintain sample related data.

Sample Status.   The logical state of a sample, such as LOGGED, COMPLETED, and UNDER TEST.

Source.   The origin of a sample. Source can be a person, place, process stream, etc.

Subroutine.   Computer programs which logically exists within a larger, "mainline" program. Subroutines are used to modularize a computer program.

Tailoring.   Small modifications to a computer program or computer system, such as a LIMS.

Test.   Taken collectively, a series of steps performed to analyze a sample for a particular set of physical and/or analytical properties. "Test" and "method" can usually be used interchangeably.

Test Group.   A predefined set of tests.

Test Status.   The logical state of a test, such as CANCELED, FAILED, and PASSED.

Worklist.   A list of samples and assigned tests. "Worklist" and "Worksheet" can usually be used interchangeably; however, sometimes differences do exist, mainly in how the samples are sorted.

Worksheet.   See "Worklist".

Appendix C-1

User Event Routine (UER) for DEC LIMS/SM LOGIN Function

The following UER represents a customization for the manual sample LOGIN function. As noted in the first line of actual code, it is a function subroutine. The UER subroutine's name is UER_MLOGIN. The purpose of the customization is to obtain additional information from a user submitting a sample for either DSC, DTA, TGA, or TMA.

As we see, the UER does actual work only when UER_MODE = 1, which is at the pre-COMMIT point of the sample LOGIN function. The UER function status is set to "2" in the statement "UER_MODE = 2." If the sample submitter decides to abort processing or if an error is detected by the UER, the UER_MODE status of "2" will abort the database commit and cause a rollback. The UER will allow the database commit by setting the function status to "1" if no problems are detected.

```
C
C Module Name: UER_MLOGIN
C File Name:    UER_MLOGIN.FOR
C
C Author/Date: RICHARD MAHAFFEY, Computer Applications
C Lab,
C 8-NOV-1986
C
C Description: This is the UER for Manual Sample Login.
C        If the sample test code is DSC, DTA, TGA or TMA
C        then a subroutine is called to obtain more
C        information on the test requirements using FMS
C        screens.The data is stored in
C        LIMS$DATA:THERMAL_DATA.DAT for later use by
C        DRA's and UER's.
C
C        After getting the request info from the user,
C        the SAMPLE_ID, ALIQUOT_ID and CROSSREFERENCE
C        NUMBER are written to
C        LIMS$DATA:THERMAL_REQ.QUE1. This
C        information is used by PGMPTHERMAL.EXE to print
C        the Thermal Analysis Request Report for the
C        Thermal Lab.
```

245

```
C
C
C
C Revision History:
C  Date           Initials      Description
C  ------         --------      ------------------------------------
C  1/29/87        RCS           Added subroutines for DRA, TGA,
C                                 and TMA
C  2/11/87        RCS           Added code to write to
C                                 HERMAL_REQ.QUE1
C  2/16/88        RCS           Added code to call SUB_PPLANT when
C                                 UORL
C
C
C --------< Source Code Starts Here   >----------
C  INTEGER*4 FUNCTION UER_MLOGIN(SAMPLE_ID,NEW_FLAG,UER_
C  MODE)
C  IMPLICIT NONE
C
C          Variable Definitions
C
          INTEGER*4 UER_MODE,DSCCOUNT,TGACOUNT,
    #     DTACOUNT,TMACOUNT
C
    LOGICAL*1 CANCEL
C
    CHARACTER     LINE_TYPE_CHAR
    CHARACTER*15 SAMPLE_ID
    CHARACTER*1   NEW_FLAG
    CHARACTER*15 USER_ID
C
C                 Common Definitions
C
    COMMON /MLOGIN_USERID/ USER_ID
C
C
C
C------< Executable Code Starts Here   >--------
C
C
C---
C  Invoke the LIMSSM database.
C---
    INVOKE (SCHEMA = 'LIMSSM$SCHEMA',
   1 SUBSCHEMA = LIMS_SM_SS,
   2 DATABASE = LIMSSM$DATABASE:LIMSSMSC,
```

```
  3 STREAM = 1 )

    IF (UER_MODE .NE. 1) RETURN
C
    READY(CONCURRENT,RETRIEVAL)! READY THE DATABASE
    UER_MLOGIN = 2     !CAUSE ROLLBACK

C.....FIND SAMPLE_ID IN DATABASE

    FIND(FIRST,RECORD=SAMPLES,SET=ALL_SAMPLES,
  1 WHERE=SAM_SAMPLE_ID .EQ. SAMPLE_ID,
  2 END=2000)

    GET(RECORD=SAMPLES) SAM_REQUISITION_NUMBER,
  # SAM_DATE_DUE,
  # SAM_ACCOUNT_NUMBER

C.....FIND ALIQUOTS
    FIND(FIRST,RECORD=ALIQUOTS,SET=SAMPLE_ALIQUOTS,
  2 END=300)

        GO TO 195
C
  190     FIND(NEXT,RECORD=ALIQUOTS,SET=SAMPLE_ALIQUOTS,
    2     END=300)
C
  195     GET(RECORD=ALIQUOTS) ALI_ALIQUOT_ID
          DSCCOUNT = 0        !INI DSC REQUEST COUNT
          TGACOUNT = 0        !INI TGA REQUEST COUNT
          TMACOUNT = 0        !INI TMA REQUEST COUNT
          DTACOUNT = 0        !INI DTA REQUEST COUNT

C.....FIND TEST REQUESTS

    FIND(FIRST,RECORD=TEST_REQUESTS,
  1 SET=ALIQUOT_TEST_REQUESTS,
  1 END=190)
    GO TO 210

  200     FIND(NEXT,RECORD=TEST_REQUESTS,
  1 SET=ALIQUOT_TEST_REQUESTS,    1 END=190)

  210     GET(RECORD=TEST_REQUESTS) TRQ_TEST_CODE

          IF(TRQ_TEST_CODE .EQ. 'DSC')GO TO 220
          IF(TRQ_TEST_CODE .EQ. 'DTA')GO TO 230
```

```
          IF(TRQ_TEST_CODE .EQ. 'TGA')GO TO 240
          IF(TRQ_TEST_CODE .EQ. 'TMA')GO TO 250
          IF(TRQ_TEST_CODE .EQ. 'UORL') GOTO 260
          GO TO 200              ! NEXT TEST CODE

C.....FOUND DSC
C.....DISPLAY DSC SPECIFIC FORM AND GET DATA FROM
C     SUBMITTER,
C   WRITE DSC SPECIFIC DATA TO FILE
C LIMS$DATA:THERMAL_DATA.DAT

220  CALL SUB_DSC_SPECIFIC_DATA(CANCEL,SAMPLE_ID,
   1 ALI_ALIQUOT_ID,DSCCOUNT,SAM_REQUISITION_NUMBER,
   2 USER_ID)
     IF(CANCEL .EQ..TRUE.)GO TO 2000! USER WANT TO CANCEL?
     GO TO 200          ! NEXT TEST CODE

C.....FOUND DTA
C.....DISPLAY DTA SPECIFIC FORM AND GET DATA FROM
C     SUBMITTER,
C     WRITE DTA SPECIFIC DATA TO FILE
C     LIMS$DATA:THERMAL_DATA.DAT
230 DTACOUNT = DTACOUNT + 1
     CALL SUB_DTA_SPECIFIC_DATA(CANCEL,SAMPLE_ID,
   1 ALI_ALIQUOT_ID,DTACOUNT,SAM_REQUISITION_NUMBER,
   2 USER_ID)
     IF(CANCEL .EQ. .TRUE.)GO TO 2000! USER WANT TO CANCEL?
     GO TO 200          ! NEXT TEST CODE

C.....FOUND TGA
C.....DISPLAY TGA SPECIFIC FORM AND GET DATA FROM
C     SUBMITTER,
C   WRITE TGA SPECIFIC DATA TO FILE
C LIMS$DATA:THERMAL_DATA.DAT

240 TGACOUNT = TGACOUNT + 1
     CALL SUB_TGA_SPECIFIC_DATA(CANCEL,SAMPLE_ID,
   1 ALI_ALIQUOT_ID,TGACOUNT,SAM_REQUISITION_NUMBER,
   2 USER_ID)
     IF(CANCEL .EQ. .TRUE.)GO TO 2000! USER WANT TO CANCEL?
     GO TO 200          ! NEXT TEST CODE

C.....FOUND TMA
C.....DISPLAY TMA SPECIFIC FORM AND GET DATA FROM
C     SUBMITTER,
C   WRITE TMA SPECIFIC DATA TO FILE
C LIMS$DATA:THERMAL_DATA.DAT
```

```
250 TMACOUNT = TMACOUNT + 1
    CALL SUB_TMA_SPECIFIC_DATA(CANCEL,SAMPLE_ID,
  1 ALI_ALIQUOT_ID,TMACOUNT,SAM_REQUISITION_NUMBER,
  2 USER_ID)
    IF(CANCEL .EQ. .TRUE.)GO TO 2000! USER WANT TO CANCEL?
    GO TO 200           ! NEXT TEST CODE
C—
C   We have a sample logged for UORL, call the subroutine
C     to get
C   the request info and write it to the file.
C—

 260 CALL SUB_PPLANT(CANCEL,SAMPLE_ID,
     # SAM_DATE_DUE,
     # SAM_ACCOUNT_NUMBER,SAM_REQUISITION_NUMBER)
     IF(CANCEL .EQ. .TRUE.) GO TO 2000 ! USER CANCEL?

 300      UER_MLOGIN = 1 ! EVERYTHING OK — CAUSE COMMIT

2000      IF(CANCEL) THEN
              IF(DSCCOUNT .GT. 0 .OR. DTACOUNT .GT. 0 .OR.
     #            TGACOUNT .GT. 0 .OR. TMACOUNT .GT. 0) THEN
          CALL
     #   DELETE_THERMAL_REQ(SAMPLE_ID,ALI_ALIQUOT_ID,
     #            SAM_REQUISITION_NUMBER)
         END IF
        END IF
        RETURN
          END
```

Appendix C-2

User Action Routine (UAR) for DEC LIMS/SM Review Test Results Function

The following UAR represents customization of the "Action Code" field of the forms associated with the *review test results* functions — "review test results by sample" (shown in Figure 8-3), "review test results by test code," and "review test results by worksheet." The UAR's name is UAR_REVIEW. UAR_REVIEW is called every time a LIMS user enters a response into the *action code* field. This UAR's purpose is to invoke an automatic test result reporting mechanism. When the user enters an "A" into the field, indicating that the test result displayed on that line is approved, the UAR reads some data from the form (sample ID, aliquot ID, test code, and run number) and writes them to a file. A separate program is then executed to extract the test results for the sample from the database and send them to the user. Thus, by just entering "A" in the action code field of the review test results form, the user approves the results and sends the report in one simple step.

```
C          L I M S   FORTRAN Module
C Module Name: UAR_REVIEW
C File Name:   UAR_REVIEW.FOR
C
C Author/Date: Richard Siggins    3/12/87
C
C Description: This FMS UAR runs on ACTION_CODE field on
C     forms REVIEW1S, REVIEW1W, and REVIEW1T to get
C     the SAMPLE_ID, ALIQUOT_ID, TEST_CODE and
C     RUN_NUMBER and store this info in a common area.
C     SEND_RESULTS will use this info to send the
C     results out to the submitters.
C
C Related FMS Forms:
C     REVIEW1S, REVIEW1W, REVIEW1T
C
C——< Source Code Starts Here >———
C
```

```
INTEGER*4 FUNCTION UAR_REVIEW
IMPLICIT NONE
C
C
C                 Parameter Definitions
C
PARAMETER      ARRAY_SIZE = 75
C
C                 Variable Definitions
C
INTEGER*4   NO_ENTRIES C
CHARACTER*15
  # SAMPLE_ID,STORED_SAMPLE_IDS(ARRAY_ SIZE)
CHARACTER*4
  # ALIQUOT_ID,STORED_ALIQUOT_IDS(ARRAY_SIZ)
CHARACTER*10
  # TEST_CODE,STORED_TEST_CODES(ARRAY_ SIZE)
CHARACTER*5
  # RUN_NUMBER,STORED_RUN_NUMBERS(ARRAY_SIZ)

   CHARACTER*2    TEST_STATUS
   CHARACTER*1    ACTION_CODE
C
C                 |Common Statements|
C
   COMMON /RCS_REVIEW/ NO_ENTRIES,STORED_SAMPLE_IDS,
   #        STORED_ALIQUOT_IDS,STORED_TEST_CODES,
   #        STORED_RUN_NUMBERS
C
C
C                 Data Definitions
C
   DATA NO_ENTRIES /0/
C
C
C                 Include Structures
C
C
   INCLUDE 'LIMS$SOURCE:DML_FDVDEF.FOR'
C
C
C————-<  Executable Code Starts Here  >————
C
C
C
   UAR_REVIEW = FDV$K_UVAL_SUC
   type *,'entering UAR_REVIEW'
```

```
C—
C  If the action code is A (approve) then
C  determine the SAMPLE_ID, ALIQUOT_ID, TEST_CODE and
C  RUN_NUMBER field values.
C—
      CALL FDV$RET (ACTION_CODE,'ACTION_CODE')
      CALL FDV$RET (TEST_STATUS,'TEST_STATUS')
      IF(ACTION_CODE.EQ.'A'.AND.TEST_STATUS.NE.'RA') THEN
        CALL FDV$RET (SAMPLE_ID,'SAMPLE_ID')
        CALL FDV$RET (ALIQUOT_ID,'ALIQUOT_ID')
        CALL FDV$RET (TEST_CODE,'TEST_CODE')
        CALL FDV$RET (RUN_NUMBER,'RUN_NUMBER')
C
      IF(NO_ENTRIES .LT. ARRAY_SIZE) THEN
        NO_ENTRIES = NO_ENTRIES + 1
        STORED_SAMPLE_IDS(NO_ENTRIES) = SAMPLE_ID
        STORED_ALIQUOT_IDS(NO_ENTRIES) = ALIQUOT_ID
        STORED_TEST_CODES(NO_ENTRIES) = TEST_CODE
        STORED_RUN_NUMBERS(NO_ENTRIES) = RUN_NUMBER
        IF(NO_ENTRIES .EQ. ARRAY_SIZE) THEN
          CALL FDV$PUTL('Writting the tests to the send '
     #            //'results queue...')
          CALL SUB_QUE_REVIEW
          NO_ENTRIES = 0
        END IF
      END IF
      END IF
C
      type *,'leaving UAR_REVIEW'
      RETURN
      END
```

Appendix C-3

Data Reduction Algorithm (DRA) for DEC LIMS/SM

The following DRA represents customization of LIMS/SM. Each time a test result is entered for a particular specific test, this DRA executes. The name of the DRA is "DRA_ASH." As the program listing shows, the routine merely "RE-TURN"s each time when the first three values are entered. When the fourth value is entered, the routine first defines default values for the three components, "TEMP," "CRUC_TYPE," and "ASH_TYPE," which will be displayed on the screen upon RETURN. It then calculates the "%ASH" final result, which is also displayed on the screen.

"DRA_ASH" is a very simple DRA. Some DRAs may present additional screens for the user to fill in. Others perform an instrument data transfer or read data from a file already transferred from an instrument. Complicated screening of the values keyed in by the user is possible using a DRA. Database searches and access to other software systems could also be included if necessary. "DRA_ASH" is typical in that it does calculate the final result, but it could have been made to do anything.

```
C*******************************************************
C
CYYY  Determination of Oxide and Sulfate Ash
CC******************************************************
      INTEGER*4 FUNCTION DRA_ASH(CODES$,VALUES$)

      INTEGER CODE,VALUE,OTS$CVT_T_F,I,J,K
      INCLUDE '($SSDEF)'
      CHARACTER*(*) CODES$
      CHARACTER*(10) COMCODES$(8),VALUES$(8)
      CHARACTER*(10) COMPONENTS$(8)
      INTEGER POSITION(8),COMPONENTS
      REAL VALUES(8)

      PARAMETER
     1 TARE_WGT=1,GROSS_WGT=2,FINAL_WGT=3,NO_CYCLES=4,
     2 TEMP=5,CRUC_TYPE=6,ASH_TYPE=7,PCT_ASH=8

      PARAMETER BLANKS='    '
```

```
DATA COMPONENTS$/'TARE_WGT ','GROSS_WGT
#','FINAL_WGT ',
1'NO_CYCLES ','TEMP','CRUC_TYPE ',
2       'ASH_TYPE ','%ASH'/

  DRA_ASH=2          !sets function to failure

  COMPONENTS=LEN(CODES$)/10
  DO I=1,COMPONENTS
   J=1+10*(I-1)
   K=10*I
   COMCODES$(I)=CODES$(J:K)
  END DO

  DO VALUE=1,8
   POSITION(VALUE)=0
   DO CODE=1,COMPONENTS
     IF(COMCODES$(CODE).EQ.COMPONENTS$(VALUE)) THEN
     POSITION(VALUE)=CODE
     IF((VALUE.NE.CRUC_TYPE.AND.VALUE.NE.
1    ASH_TYPE).AND.
2      OTS$CVT_T_F(VALUES$(CODE),VALUES(VALUE),
3      %VAL(0),%VAL(0),%VAL(1)).NE.SS$_NORMAL)
4      RETURN
    END IF
   END DO
  END DO
  DRA_ASH=1          !sets function to success
   IF((POSITION(TARE_WGT).NE.0).AND.
1    (VALUES$(POSITION(TARE_WGT)).NE.BLANKS))
2    THEN
     IF((POSITION(GROSS_WGT).NE.0).AND.
1    (VALUES$(POSITION(GROSS_WGT)).NE.BLANKS))
2    THEN
     IF((POSITION(FINAL_WGT).NE.0).AND.
1      (VALUES$(POSITION(FINAL_WGT)).NE.BLANKS))
2       THEN
       IF((POSITION(NO_CYCLES).NE.0).AND.
1        (VALUES$(POSITION(NO_CYCLES)).NE.BLANKS))
2         THEN
            IF(VALUES(NO_CYCLES).GT.0) THEN

     IF(VALUES$(POSITION(TEMP)).EQ.''    )
1     THEN
       VALUES$(POSITION(TEMP))='600'
     END IF
```

```
      IF(VALUES$(POSITION(CRUC_TYPE)).EQ.'')
1     THEN
        VALUES$(POSITION(CRUC_TYPE))='PORCELAIN '
      END IF
      IF(VALUES$(POSITION(ASH_TYPE)).EQ.''      )
1     THEN
        VALUES$(POSITION(ASH_TYPE))='OXIDE'
      END IF

   VALUES(PCT_ASH)=((VALUES(FINAL_WGT)-
1     VALUES(TARE_WGT))*100.0)/
2     (VALUES(GROSS_WGT)-VALUES(TARE_WGT))

      ENCODE(10,100,VALUES$(POSITION(PCT_ASH)))
1                 VALUES(PCT_ASH)

      ELSE
   DRA_ASH=2          !sets function to failure

         END IF
        END IF
       END IF
      END IF
     END IF

     RETURN
100  FORMAT(F10.2)
     END
```

Index